WE
CAN
DO
THIS!

Adult Children and Aging Parents Planning for Success

Lorraine (Lorrie) Morales

L. Morales

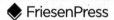
FriesenPress

Suite 300 - 990 Fort St
Victoria, BC, V8V 3K2
Canada

www.friesenpress.com

Dedication to my parents: Fred and Ruby Judin

Some of the names of individual in the stories have been changed in order to protect their identity. Any resulting resemblance to persons living or dead is entirely coincidental and unintentional.

ISBN
978-1-5255-5811-5 (Hardcover)
978-1-5255-5812-2 (Paperback)
978-1-5255-5813-9 (eBook)

1. FAMILY & RELATIONSHIPS, ELDERCARE

Distributed to the trade by The Ingram Book Company

Sure, you can go on the internet and find thousands of sites dealing with "What to do when you're in a crisis." But what if you had a plan in place beforehand to deal with that situation?

What if you were proactive and had preplanned your loved one's quality of life in his or her later years, or even had some help for yourself? After all, we are the adults!

How much better would that make your life, and the lives of others? What about even saving time? That's where this book will serve as a guide to help direct your decisions about a plan. I know that I sure could have used one many months ago … before we laid my parents to rest.

ACKNOWLEDGEMENTS

Thanks to my brothers and sisters who have gone through this with me, and to my "tribe" of supporters, encouragers, readers, contributors, and all those who have been, are, or will be going through all of this and more. Love keeps me and all of us together.

DEDICATION

To my parents—Fred and Ruby Judin

PREFACE

Sure, you can go on the internet and find thousands of sites dealing with "What to do when you're in a crisis." You can research facts and information about nearly any topic on the planet. And while our intentions for the care of our loved ones are generally heartfelt and sincere, many of us don't consider the topic of aging until we're either in the middle of a situation or faced with decisions that need to be made in the best interests of those we love. But what if you had a plan in place beforehand to deal with those issues? There are countless families, including mine, who have had to consider various aspects of caregiving.

Because I was part of that large group looking for cost effective yet comfortable, manageable facilities and care for my parents in the last years of their lives, I had to consider many options to ensure they received proper care, both at home and elsewhere. My siblings and I had to understand not just our well-being, but that of our parents. We had to learn how to navigate the various issues of housing, finances, legalities, and communication—even though we were somewhat organized.

We learned many facts, understood many issues, and solved many problems as we ventured through the ocean of caregiving. Sometimes the direction and decisions were very clear, such as Mom spending her last days in a hospice. At other times, we were at a loss as to what our next steps should be, like when Dad ended up in the hospital and needed more care. These are the lessons were learned. But …

What if you were proactive and specifically planned your loved one's quality of life in his or her later years, or even had some help for yourself? After all, we are the adults!

How much better would that make your life, and the lives of others? What about even saving time?

You can get organized ahead of time. You can have a team of supporters to guide you on your journey as a caregiver. What if you knew about financial, legal, and funeral information before your death? What if you had a home in place when you were either healthy or failing in health? Each of us will certainly have some role to play in eldercare during our lifetime. That's where this book will serve as a guide to help direct your decisions about a plan. I know that I sure could have used one many months ago … before we laid my parents to rest.

It's also not a huge revelation that all of us are going to age differently. Ageism impacts society. One day, each of us will have his or her turn to navigate the waters of aging.

It's also not a secret that many of us don't want to dwell on the topic of aging, as that could cause a possible discussion of our vulnerability and mortality. Not only are our fears focused on this, but we also have other fears about aging besides the physical deterioration of our bodies, such as financial worries.

There are cases in which the price for private senior care is often prohibitive. An example of this is a group in Langley, British Columbia, who were inspired by a facility in the Netherlands by opening a village for the elderly, focusing on dementia patients.[1] The cost to live there is expensive, with a price tag of $70,000–$90,000 annually, or $195–$245/day. I know that my parents would never have been able to afford to live there, nor would many others. Although at one point in my dad's life it would have been a blessing because of his dementia.

Before we can adequately address the growth of the senior segment of our society, we have to understand the need for adequate care and attention for our loved ones on many levels and at a variety of price points. I'm certainly more aware of my own need for future care and, as a result of my experiences, decided to write this book for caregiving to make sense for me and others.

As many as 8.1 million Canadians, or 50 per cent of caregivers, care for a parent, in-law, or another person.[2] Individuals, couples, and families going through similar caregiving circumstances ask: "How did this suddenly happen to me?"

When I meet with people both personally and professionally from my generation, the discussion steers to the topic of the elderly, our aging parents and loved ones, and I realize that I am only one of thousands who have suddenly been given the title of "caregiver." It wasn't just about me and my job, kids, family, and friends, but about my parents as well. And I ask, "Why me?"

When my friend Trish and I met recently, we shared our frustrating moments and similar circumstances. Because we're caught between caring for our families and ourselves and having to care for our elderly parents, we fall into the "vice grip" category. She gathered countless resources and I started writing. By discussing ideas about what was working for us and what wasn't, we thought that sharing information, helping others, and guiding them on this journey would be in our best interest. Thus, the inception of a book, one that could be shared with others, read in random chapter order, and passed on to our caregivers when "our time has come."

The book was written for Canadians, specifically Albertans, but some of it will be applicable to those in other countries. I encourage people to research what's available where they live, as terminology, laws, medical services, or housing will likely be different.

When I was visiting my father at his seniors' home, the manager and I had a conversation about caregiving. He asked me to check out his sister, Deb's, story. [3]

Debbie Cook shared her story at last year's Palliative Care Conference in Calgary (2017). I met with her recently, and she reassured me that there is a need for information in layman's terms to assist the caregiver. These experiences are our personal stories. What's yours?

This information isn't a revelation, and it shouldn't be considered legal advice, as only a lawyer can provide this based on your circumstances; however, I hope the real stories resonate with you and that the helpful websites, tips, and resources make life easier when caring for the aged—after all, we've been given a huge responsibility with the title of "caregiver."

As I look back on my journey, I see that the experiences, memories, and moments spent with my parents mattered. Much of my book is based on time spent with my father, because when my mother passed away, I realized just how much care she had given to my dad. So, say a little prayer and put a plan put into place!

My dad, sitting in his La-Z-Boy, commented to me as I reached down to tie up his runners: "Bet you didn't think you'd ever have to tie my shoes, help me to the bathroom, or sit with me by my hospital bed."

That was the evening before the ambulance took Dad to the hospital after his fall at the seniors' residence, when he sliced his ear open and fractured his pelvis.

I said, "No, Dad, I always thought you and Mom would be around forever, never getting old."

My parents were practical, organized, energetic adults who never stopped parenting, even when I was fifty-nine years old. "You work too hard," they'd say when I'd pop over for a visit on my way home from work. "The speed limit is only thirty through this school zone," they'd exclaim as I'd drive them to an appointment.

"I'll be telling you what to do until the day I die," my mom used to say. And when she did die, reality struck. Mom had been diagnosed with cancer two times previous to her final bone cancer diagnosis. In some ways, I think we thought she'd beat the disease again. That didn't happen.

The tables were turned upside down, and I suddenly became the caregiver for my dad—the man who'd been married to my mother for over sixty-one years. That's how old I was when I became the "caregiver."

The role reversal was odd, because my husband and I had already raised our two sons. I was semi-retired, ready to travel and adhere to my own schedule and routines. I truly loved my dad and wanted to treat him with the dignity he deserved and honor him as my father, not just some old man in a seniors' home. I now had to devote time to him, because his world had been turned upside down too.

"Dad, did you go to the bathroom?" I'd often ask before we'd head into the city for an appointment. I felt like the parent; he was the child.

Through caring for both of my parents up until their deaths, I've learned much about patience, about my parents and my family, and mostly about myself. Perhaps it's time to share my story to help others along the journey, should you be dealing with aging parents now or in the future.

Many people have experiences of caregiving, and their advice needs to be recognized. Most of us have a story to tell or have listened to someone else's story.

Even though our experiences are all different, every caregiver I have met has had the same doubt: "I'm not sure I can do this!" I wrote this book to assure you that you can do it, and I can show you how. You do not have to do this alone. Our goal is very similar: how to care—or rather, prepare—for caregiving? Those are our stories. We can do this! I'll say a little prayer for you!

INTRODUCTION

"It's not the load that breaks you down, it's the way you carry it."
Lou Holtz [4]

After a full career, I retired from teaching. I was simply living life, working on a few contracts, and guest teaching the odd day. I was reluctant to think that my parents needed anything but a quick visit or phone call every few days or weeks, as they were quite self-sufficient. This is the experience of many people who have elderly parents who are still fairly independent.

Often, I would pop by their condo because I lived close, and as some of them lived out of province, my other siblings would check up with a weekly phone call. My brothers lived nearby, but I was the eldest daughter, retired, and had more time on my hands to devote to ensuring Mom and Dad were doing all right. After all, we recognized they were aging.

Just after my retirement, we started noticing a few red flags, so we'd get together for family visits, chat on the phone weekly, and have family conversations. Fortunately, we were a fairly healthy, functioning family. We were able to talk about any issue we felt was important. The main topic of conversation was revolved around how we

LORRAINE (LORRIE) MORALES

were going to take care of Mom and Dad as they aged and declined in health?

Mom would say, "Your dad put his socks in the dishwasher the other day," or "He was up at 5:00 a.m., dressed and ready to go threshing." Mom would document Dad's dementia progression over the years in her journals, and we would ask her if we needed to start searching for a place at a memory care facility. She'd reply, "Not yet."

According to Statistics Canada's website, almost half (48 per cent) of caregivers reported giving care to their own parents or parents-in-law in 2012. [5]

Adult children like myself were almost four times more likely to report caring for a parent, and 2.5 times more likely to report caring for their own mother than father. I was the opposite of that by caring for my dad. We always believed Mom would outlive Dad, but we had just celebrated dad's 86th birthday!

It's easy for life to get in the way of tough conversations or planning ahead for struggles that seem far away. As my peers and I get older, I hear more stories about family members wondering, "What do I do now?" I didn't realize at the time that I was one of many adult children finding herself caring for her parent. And I certainly was not prepared for any part of it.

As Gaye Warthe, Ph.D. and Associate Dean of Teaching and Learning at Mount Royal University in Calgary, Alberta says, "*To be prudent, families need to start having these conversations early on.*" [6]

Why do people balk at change until a crisis forces change? Why wait until catastrophes arise or a loved one dies or we're in a crisis? It **is** possible to be prepared for most things. Before I go on any journey, I often plan the trip and equip myself for where I want to go. I get organized and then enjoy the ride on a less bumpy road. Heavens, I even have Google maps to help me out these days! Why not follow this process when considering the care of our loved ones?

Let's celebrate life and make the moments with our loved ones matter, so that we can also make happy memories with these valued family and friends. Let's also gather the right tools and equipment to guide us in preparing for the care of these loved ones, so that we can have less stress in our lives as well. Health Canada tells us that the leading cause of many of our diseases is stress related. If we took more preventative action, what else might happen? Would we gain more and better time with the people we love?

> "It's funny. I always imagined when I was a kid that adults always had some kind of inner toolbox full of shining tools: the saw of discernment, the hammer of wisdom, the sandpaper of patience. But when I grew up, I found that life handed you these bent old tools—friendship, prayer, conscience, honesty—and said—'Do the best you can with these—they will have to do. And mostly, against all odds— they do.'" Anne Lamott - Traveling Mercies—Some Thoughts on Faith [7]

I suppose that nothing really prepares us for the moments when we do fall apart; regardless of the tools we have in our toolbox. I remember clearly the day I hit the wall. Being the eldest, having it "all together," and being strong for everyone else was always part of my character, so when it happened, everyone was surprised at my falling apart.

I was moving Dad's things from his and Mom's condo to an independent living facility in my town outside of the city. I was also visiting my cancer-filled mom at the hospice in the city, managing their finances, and taking care of their life changes. I was contacting and informing family, relatives, and friends about what was going on, and meeting with the landlady and the women's group from my parents' church. I had to drive my sister to the airport, text my brother to pick up medications for my father, and I hadn't even thought about what I was going to have for supper when, and if, I even returned at a decent hour. Everyone around me seemed oblivious and busy with their own worlds and lives when it hit me: "I am in the middle of my parents' lives, and I didn't even sign up for this!"

I had no training! What was I supposed to do? The tears fell, and I came to an abrupt moment of feeling like I'd hit a wall. I was sitting in my SUV in a parking lot overlooking the river. The greasy burger I was eating was dripping down my arm, and I reached for the take-out napkins to wipe my tears. I grabbed my sunglasses off the dash and put them on so that anyone walking by wouldn't notice my tear-stained face. As I opened the window to divert the onion smell into the fresh air, I knew that regardless of my sorrow, suffering, or struggles, I was going to love and care for my parents at this age and stage in their lives. I also talked to God and asked Him to give me the strength I needed to do it. Saying a little prayer helped me through.

I was in high stress mode while trying to make sense of everything that was going on around me. Not a great place to be, but I did have some bent old tools in my box.

Thankfully, I had faith and loving family and friends who supported and understood me. I had understanding and compassionate employers and a community that stepped forward to help. I could be open and honest and share those feelings with the people in my life.

That night I drove home under a beautiful full moon. When I arrived in the house, I called my sisters. They told me to do what I could, that they loved me and were praying for me, and to not do it all.

They'd be in a car headed to my house or on the next plane the minute I needed them.

What a blessing!

Becoming a caregiver can be thrust upon you gradually or very suddenly. For me, it was gradual. I didn't often get to choose what happened, but I learned that I could choose how to react to what was happening. Still, I regularly felt overwhelmed by all I was managing, an experience you might be having right now.

In addition to being a caregiver for your loved ones, you may also have jobs and other commitments. Some days will feel like you're caught in the middle of all that's going on; hence, "the sandwich generation," or as I put it, "the vice grip"—a fitting title for so many of us caught in the middle of caregiving and the pressure on us to do the job.

Like me, you may also be thinking, "I have no training! What am I supposed to do?" Believe it or not, there are colleges that teach courses on being a caregiver. Programs exist to provide care for the caregivers as well. Seminars, training programs and courses qualify you to become certified as a caregiver. I never had the paper certificate, but I was certainly trying to handle all the roles of a caregiver with limited knowledge, credentials, or qualifications. I also decided that I was not going to beat myself up over how I was performing in a role that wasn't going to last a lifetime. And don't worry … I'm not going to encourage you to go get training. I wrote this book so that you wouldn't have to.

Looking back on the whole experience of caring for my parents, after having been through that falling apart moment and, to some degree, still going through parts of it, I understand how taking on all of that responsibility has affected my personal life and health, my coping and organizational skills, my work, and my relationships with others. That's not even mentioning time management. The fact of the matter was and is … I am a caregiver! And that role has changed me.

Rosalynn Carter, former First Lady of United States of America, once said, "*There are only four kinds of people in this world: those who have been caregivers; those who are currently caregivers; those who will be caregivers and those who will need caregivers.*"[8]

Sometimes, caregivers are individuals who provide care and assistance, without pay, for family members and friends in need of support. They're caring because of physical, cognitive, or mental health conditions. That was me.

On the other hand, caregivers can be professionals who are trained to do what they do. Some are hired privately and paid to provide services. That's their career. Some of these individuals love their job, and you can tell by their work. Be sure to have these types of caregivers in your loved ones' lives.

Both types of caregivers are there to assist, reassure, comfort, and care for other human beings. They want to make life a bit easier for those they're caring for, a task that becomes more layered when those people are friends or family.

When you're caring for your parents, you don't want to think of them only as cancer or dementia patients (nor should you); you want to help them along their journey as individuals who are valued and loved. To do this, I had to learn patience, communicate my feelings, and let go of what I couldn't control. I had to count my blessings and remember at times to breathe, because there were times when I had to bite my tongue and hold my breath!

Before Mom and Dad required full-time care, when they'd moved closer to family in the last five years of their lives, my mother was still driving—but sitting in the passenger seat made me a bit nervous. Dad had given up his driver's license years before, but Mom wanted her independence, and she had that with the car. They struggled at times with getting the groceries and Dad's walker into their vehicle and up to the condo, and I realized that, eventually, the toll on their strength and the trying of Mom's patience with Dad had become too much.

Eventually, Mom started letting go of a few things as well. She allowed my brother to pick up the groceries, and my sister in law or myself to drive her to some of her appointments and do a little of the housekeeping. Our backs were a little stronger!

Mom loved to share her recipes and to cook and bake, but standing in the kitchen became tiring. Dad, on the other hand, was a safety hazard in that space. When he almost dumped a pot of boiling water on himself when he slipped by the stove, we outlawed him from cooking at all. Housekeeping became onerous, and with all the jobs of day-to-day living becoming difficult for our parents, we as siblings collectively decided to get assistance from others, and we had lots of questions. Where do we start? Who do we contact? Where do we go from here? Is there a right way to go about all of this?

If you already think of yourself as the caregiver, with a thousand questions to get answered, then you're on the right path. Asking questions is the first, and sometimes the hardest, step. Even if you don't consider yourself a caregiver but have been given the task, this book will help you ask the questions you need to ask, and to figure out the answers that make sense for you and your family. This book includes stories (mine and others') of mistakes and successes. In each chapter, the destinations along the journey of caregiving include:

- Where to live based on health needs
- Building a team to communicate with and connect to for emotional support
- Understanding legalities
- Discovering financial stability
- Staying well—emotionally, spiritually, physically, and socially
- Different types of housing for the aged
- The final days
- Reflections
- Resources

You'll find tips, advice, and discovered knowledge that will save you time, help keep you sane and organized, and simplify your life in the midst of caregiving and, at times, chaos. You'll find guidance to plan ahead or to put a plan in action right now if you need to.

There are a million reasons to put this off. I know.

But I don't have time! Heard that one before? Or how about …

I would, but …

Or …

I tried, but it didn't work.

Or …

We thought about it, but …

This book is your chance to say "No more excuses" and to get out of the "vice grip" so you can get going and be free to try these ideas.

Are you ready for the first step on this journey? It's okay if you're not. I'll be right there with you. Read on. We can do this! I just said a little prayer for you.

CHAPTER 1:
STAYING ORGANIZED
First Steps

If you want to stay organized and sane and keep it all together, then head to the nearest store that sells file folders and files. Sit down with the papers. I'd recommend working together to file information with your parents and eventually doing it for them but keeping them informed when you do any filing. Thankfully, my sister runs her own business and got things organized, categorized, and labelled for my parents.

She had flown in from Vancouver to visit my parents one weekend and went to locate their car insurance information. Mom and Dad had a desk in their den filled with different papers. My sister was frustrated with the disorganization, so she took one of Dad's older filing cases, bought and labelled new folders with tabs, and kept the case in their office so that when any of us siblings needed to find or file any document, it was at our fingertips. This proved very helpful when I had to notify the various services when we gave up their condo.

By starting a file folder for each loved one, we were able to retrieve documents and information quickly. Even if your parents are together, keep each individual's information separate. You'll be glad you did when there's an emergency. That way, you can just grab the file—it's much easier than sifting through a ream of papers stuck at the bottom of a kitchen drawer or old filing cabinet.

It's also a great idea to get a folder started for yourself, as a reminder that eventually you'll need to get all your papers in order. Find a safe place that trusted individuals can locate when they need to look at your information. Make a list.

You can have as many file tabs as you want, but the folders listed below are the ones I found most helpful and useful for information I needed to have at my fingertips.

- medical history and medications
- SIN number and income tax forms
- Personal Directive and Power of Attorney (DNR)
- wills
- passports
- birth/marriage/divorce/adoption certificates
- bank statements and investments
- credit cards
- PIN numbers for accounts
- bills (cable TV, telephone, power, water, taxes, gas, etc.)
- vehicle information and insurance
- mortgage or rental agreement / property ownership documents (land titles)
- list of jewellery, collectibles, furniture items
- medical equipment or supplies and receipts

- list of phone contacts (private and business) and emails
- passwords for email, credit cards, bank debit card, accounts
- church directory
- club Memberships
- accountant
- gun registry or collection information
- magazine or other subscriptions
- list of assets (trailers, snowmobiles, recreation toys, boats) with serial numbers
- pets
- other

Some people want to create word documents or download forms (PDF) on the computer and store them in folders on their desk or laptops for quick reference or access. If this is the case, be sure to save information on a thumb drive or other exterior drive, and always make a hard copy for the file folder.

Another useful tip is to get yourself a small, portable binder or folder to take to medical and other appointments. Keep a calendar and medical or legal information in that folder. A little notepad or sticky notes are useful for jotting down important information from the visit. You can sort things out after the appointment.

For example, after I'd get home after dropping Mom off, I'd call my siblings or email them to explain what the doctor had said. I was always thankful to have my notes with me to help explain what had transpired.

When caretaking, you'll likely need to record conversations, write down contacts, or collect business cards for future reference. Buy plastic sleeves for a binder in which to keep the contacts, tape the cards into a notebook for easy reference, or put them in a sleeve in a binder or notebook. Make notes, lists, and record doctors' instructions. This is handy when referencing or communicating information to siblings and family. We always think we're going to remember everything, but the smallest of details can be lost or forgotten when you're concerned and occupied with a parent. Often after an oncologist's appointment with Mom I'd forget the names of some of her medications, even as we were leaving the parking lot.

Dad had hydrocephalus. The way I mentally noted that prognosis was by thinking of water seeping out of our pores, but I still had to write it down to remember. We often had to go up to the clinic to have him reassessed, with follow-ups on a quarterly basis. One day he was sitting at my brother's for lunch with my mother, Ruby, when my sister-in-law asked him, "Fred, how was your appointment last week?"

"Fabulous!" Dad replied with sarcasm in his voice. "They made me walk down the hall and look at a bunch of pictures. It doesn't do a thing for me!"

"Wow," my sister-in-law retorted. "What was the name of your doctor?"

Dad's face went blank, and you could see he was trying to remember, but couldn't. Finally, he smiled and asked, "What do you call that red stone like a diamond?"

"You mean a Ruby?"

"Yes, that's it!" Then turning to Mom, he asked, "Ruby, what's that doctor's name?"

Forgetfulness is part of all of our daily lives; however, dementia can slowly progress. We certainly saw that with my dad. He got to the point of not being cognitively aware of where he was. When he was living alone at the seniors' home, at times he'd call my brothers and I at five o'clock in the morning, asking us to pick him up from the hotel. He didn't realize the time, but we certainly did! Sometimes when we'd visit him at the seniors' home, he'd nod off to sleep every few minutes because of his vascular dementia. He'd suddenly wake up and pick up the conversation where he'd left off.

I'm thankful that we'd taken care of so many details regarding legalities, finances, and living arrangements beforehand. If we hadn't been as organized, things could have looked quite differently because of Dad's memory. Planning takes the stress off both parties, caregiver and loved ones.

Architects use it when building skyscrapers; city planners use it for new developments; and airline pilots log their flight plans. Yet when it comes to anticipating aging or talking about what's important to us in our later years, when we may be incapable of making decisions or caring for ourselves, it doesn't seem that important.

John F. Kennedy stated in the State of the Union Address on January 11,1962 that: *"The time to repair the roof is when the sun is shining."*[9] It makes sense, but we often have other commitments, business, or activities that supersede planning.

Gaye Warthe, Ph.D. from Mount Royal University, indicates that,

> *"The trauma that comes from watching a loved one decline can cause a situation rife with potential for family*

upheaval. Family members often disagree about finances, care choices, living arrangements, planning and more. The stories are myriad...Families need to be able to take time, sit down and talk about what needs to be discussed." [10]

There are multiple guides designed to help family members discuss or create a caregiving plan for aging parents or relatives, friends, neighbours, or even yourself! You could spend days on your computer just searching for those sites. There are even sections in major bookstores that deal with aging and mental health. Prioritizing planning is essential to less stress. We can do this! I did!

After reading countless books on caregiving and asking various experts, such as senior care managers and other caregivers, for advice, I realized that there could be a plan put into place to make caregiving less stressful on all parties. Easily said, but hardly ever the case. I resourced sites on the internet, copied important facts for my reference, and shared information with my family and friends. I perused bookshelves in bookstores, talked with other caregivers, and spent time in the library ... only to find that there was a wealth of information, but none of it right at my fingertips. I decided that there could be a Canadian, simplified guide to help myself and others through the important aspects of aging.

Ten years ago, Gail Sheehy, world renowned author of fifteen books, including *Passages in Caregiving—Turning Chaos into Confidence*, wrote,

> *Only in retrospect did I wonder why we hadn't talked about the inevitable: growing older, how might we face the assaults of body and mind? Who would take care of whom? How would we pay for it? North Americans tend to wait until we are too old and too sick to have decent, affordable choices for care in our golden (or rusted-out) years.*

Planning ahead is preferable—if you can face it. If you can't, you risk plunging into confusion in full crisis mode.[11]

Could people avoid this? We chose to plan.

As a family, we discussed options for Mom and Dad, talked about where to start, thought about questions we needed to ask, and researched where we could find resources to help us out. We didn't do it all at once, and we didn't have the answers to every question. We were all employed and had other responsibilities, but we made time for those discussions.

"I've done some research and found that Lifeline Medical Alert System looks like the best option for Mom and Dad in case they have a fall."

"Let's call them and set up an appointment to go over the information with them."

"One of us will have to be here to ensure that the instructions are clear and we know what's going on."

"I'm working and on call this week, so I can't."

"I'm not sure of my schedule, so I won't be able to be there."

"I'll set it up, but can you be here when then come?"

"I can."

I did this, and you can too.

No need to be discouraged—just get started with conversations that work for your family. We all have different dynamics, so be strong as an advocate for your parents and don't hesitate to be the one to

7

initiate and follow through with some necessary and sometimes tough conversations. Because I was the one with fewer work and family responsibilities, and I lived close to my parents, I was often the one who could be there for those appointments. At times my siblings and I disagreed about decisions that Mom and Dad or one of us made; however, the decisions made were in the best interest of our loved ones.

Watch for those red flags that can initiate the conversations as well. Recently, a friend of mine was relaying a red flag story about her mom and dad who were living independently at the time. Her dad would often get up in the middle of the night to cook something to eat. Meanwhile, her mom would be soundly sleeping in their bed. One night, her dad got up to cook himself a bowl of noodles. He put the pot on the stove, but instead of water, he filled it with oil. Needless to say, the pot started smoking. He grabbed the pot, which was extremely hot, burned his hand, and dropped the pot of smoking oil. The kitchen mat caught on fire. He grabbed a towel to douse the flames and went back to bed. You can imagine the look on her mom's face when she went into the kitchen the next morning to make breakfast! Not to mention her shock at seeing her husband's badly blistered hand.

My friend was instantly concerned about the safety of her parents. What if the fire hadn't gone out? What if her dad's burn had caused serious and permanent damage because he didn't have it treated immediately? What if their house had caught on fire? These are serious questions my friend contemplated. After I encouraged her to think about her parents' safety and well-being, my friend planned on having a discussion with her siblings.

Conversations about the future need to happen, and they don't always have to focus on a caregiving plan. When we started having our conversations, it was over dessert after family gatherings, and the conversations centred on what was important to Mom and Dad as they got older. They asked for our opinions about where they should live, who should get "the money" when they died, and where they wanted to be buried.

Recently, another friend asked her parents whether they would continue to live in their home or move to a retirement home. They were a bit taken aback by her question, but she did get some answers, and they have begun to address some issues. Perhaps your next visit could involve a casual conversation similar to that with the folks.

You may want to start with **Goals for the Future.** Make a list and check off those topics that apply. You can use the list below as a guide. These conversations can be very detailed or simply general exploration. Here are a few questions to demonstrate potential topics to discuss.

- Do you want to remain as independent as possible for as long as possible?
- Do you want to remain healthy and active? What will that look like?
- What hobbies or interests do you want to focus on?
- Do you want to work for as long as possible, volunteering or getting paid?
- Are there community groups you want to get involved with?
- Do you want to volunteer your time or expertise?
- Can you remain financially independent and, if not, how do we help you out?
- Do you want to take classes in something you always wanted to learn?

- Did you create an emergency list of people to contact?

- Do you want to start your own business venture with someone?

- Do you want to buy a retirement second home in Canada or abroad?

- Do you want to travel? Where to?

- Do you want to move closer to family so that we can see you more often?

- Do you want to relocate to another province for various reasons?

- Do you want to retire in another country?

- Do you have someone to help you with moving to another location?

- Can you help us children/grandchildren by sharing our lives?

- Can you think of any other goals for the future?

This list gets parents and adult children talking about the future.

My parents wanted to be very independent. They experienced house-sitting, travel, and spent a year caring for a couple with Alzheimer's disease living on a ranch. They even tried living in an assisted living facility for six months to experience what it would be like should they choose that option for the future. They sold their house to be closer to family members, namely myself. My mother's failing health eventually meant that they couldn't be as adventurous as they'd like.

My father enjoyed woodworking and would spend hours in his shop when my parents were living independently, but when they moved from their home and Dad's dementia progressed, it was also difficult (and dangerous) for him to pound a nail or run the saws and lathe. Eventually he had to resort to watching the others in the shop at their condo complex, smelling the sawdust, drinking coffee and telling tales with the other men there. Many would agree that keeping your parents in their home for as long as possible is the best option if at all possible.

Peter, a friend and colleague, recently shared his parents' journey of making the conscious decision to finally leave their "family home" of twenty years. Accessing the bathroom and bedrooms was no longer viable. They moved to a villa/duplex on a golf course, and even though they never played golf, they appreciated the yard maintenance. When they could no longer handle the yard work, they moved into a seniors' apartment with one bedroom. After his mother fell getting out of bed, and his father was unable to help her, she had to move into an assisted living facility that was connected to a facility where his father could live. His father would visit her often, eat supper with her in the dining room, and be close by.

All of the decisions had been made by them until his father had a few of his own visits to the hospital and was told he had to move into assisted living himself, but the facility was out of the city. After refusing to move twice, he finally had no choice. But he was frustrated and now lived fifty kilometres away from his wife in a small town. He did play bingo for the first time in his life, but it was a "tough go" for him. Finally, a room became available in his wife's facility, so after a few more moves, he relocated down the hall from her. She passed away soon after. That was not the end of the story, though.

Many of my colleague's siblings lived in Calgary, so they wanted their father closer to them. When that finally happened, his father wanted to "go home." His last move came five months later when he passed away and could be with his wife and Father in heaven. My friend Peter has concluded that moving was never a simple affair, as there were so many factors to consider. The family did have the best interests of their parents in mind and did research various facilities so that their parents could be together in their end years. There was planning involved in the entire process.

If your parents or loved ones are still in their home living independently, several questions should be asked regarding their home maintenance and living situation.

Here are a few questions to start thinking about:

- Is the rent or mortgage being paid?
- Who is checking on home repairs?
- Who is mowing the lawn? Housekeeping? Preparing meals?
- Are there any safety concerns?
- What about pet care?
- Who is buying the groceries?
- Are the bills being paid? Who is keeping track of financial records?
- Where is the list of family members' addresses, phone numbers, emails?
- Are they still driving?
- Who is helping out with bathing? Hygiene?
- Who is giving rides to run errands and appointments?
- Who is keeping the family informed?
- What if they need more care or adaptive devices, such as a walker or raised toilet seat?

Countless other questions are raised when we consider that getting older requires some planning.

Daren Heyland, a professor at Queen's University, is also an intensive care physician in Ontario. He says: *"There is a need to normalize and create conversations about what the end looks like, think about it and prepare for it."*[12] Some families don't consider end years, while others are met with opposition when the topic is even broached. These are sensitive issues.

When we communicate with our loved ones, the big questions are: "How do we know when to step in and how much do we take over? Is it possible to preserve their dignity and independence by other means?" This delicate balance of giving loved ones their say and the family a chance to share their opinions is much like raising children. When their safety is an issue, it's time to act on their behalf. By having those conversations, each situation will lend itself to seeing the warning signs, concerns, and decisions that will need to be made should those situations arise.

"It does not do to leave a live dragon out of your calculations, if you live near him." J.R.R. Tolkien - The Hobbit [13]

What if we could be ready for some of the changes? I was somewhat ready for my parents' declining health, because I'd heard stories from some relatives and friends who were caring for aging parents. This inspired me to help others on this journey of caregiving, but I still wasn't sure what it all entailed.

The Canadian Institute for Research indicates that the number of caregivers in our society is decreasing:

> Given the anticipated shortages of health care workers in Canada, competition for health care resources is expected

to be fierce in the coming years. To recruit and retain home support workers in all sectors, whether in voluntary, for-profit or public organizations, working conditions must be enhanced.[14]

The need to care for the elderly is rising. We still have to prepare for the future.

Whether individuals, couples, or families live in close proximity, or are provinces or countries apart, all caregivers and families are in various stages of determining what to do with our loved ones. Some individuals have been through this process, some are in the middle of "what to do now," and many will eventually get there. I have spoken to countless families, and the common theme I hear is: "How do we even begin to prepare for caregiving as our parents age?" When my parents were in my position, extended families tended to live in one area and care for each other. They would share the responsibilities of providing meals, transportation, and medical assistance, not to mention emotional support.

That was then, but this is now. Making a plan with the family and aging relatives might be a step in the right direction. Read on and adjust to your unique situation.

CHAPTER 1 TAKEAWAYS:

- ☐ Decide among your family members (or in the case of there being no family, trusted friends) who is going to take the lead to get the conversations started.

- ☐ Make a list of goals for the future. You can't decide what your loved one wants in their latter years or after death. Get them to tell you what they want.

☐ Get those file folders and start organizing all those documents.

The journey of a thousand miles begins with one step. - Lao Tzu[15]

DID YOU KNOW?

Fact: Apps and online tools for family caregivers will be widely adopted in the next five years.

Fact: Instead of thinking only about how to improve long-term caregiving services and supports, Canadians involved in aging health care will be looking for ways to prevent more people from needing them.

Fact: The percentage of the population developing Alzheimer's disease is going down, but because the population of older adults overall is growing, the absolute number of Alzheimer's cases is still on the rise.

Fact: In ten years, a "good death" will take priority over prolonging life. Check out Quality End of Life Care Coalition of Canada[16]

CHAPTER 2: PLANNING

For Caregivers and Aging Parents

My eldest son is getting married this summer. He and his fiancée are teachers and like to be well-organized. They know the importance of this from their experiences teaching in a middle school. Their wedding planning is going well, and they have acquired a venue, sent out invitations, had engagement photos taken, and completed most of their list of "to do" items by discussing their plan between themselves and with others. Planning a wedding is a celebratory event. Oftentimes, when planning for a lost family member, a funeral can be a celebration of a well-lived life. What if the planning was in place and there had been a discussion before that day?

A High River *Times* article entitled "Death Cafe—A First for High River Community" states that there is an international movement of Death Cafe events, with one being hosted in High River (a little town south of Calgary, Alberta). The Death Cafe provides opportunity for people to talk about death in a positive, safe environment. Perhaps there's a Death Cafe in your community. Why not go online and check it out? This could prove to be a valuable experience for the simple reason that others are experiencing the trepidation of having conversations pertaining to death. Other insights might be beneficial. We have support groups for many different topics. Death is one of them.

Gordon, a funeral director with Snodgrass Funeral Homes of High River, Alberta, stated that, *"quite often we meet with families who have made no plans, have no idea what their next (step) is going to be as far as dealing with death. Typically, people don't talk about it until they're in its grip."* [17]

That's where planning makes the difference and makes sense. Because caregiving is inevitable, unpredictable, and requires flexible management to benefit all parties involved, it's best to pre-plan for even the finality of death. Because we often avoid the topic of death, it's more difficult to discuss. This often happens when the family is split up and there are relational issues to be resolved, or planning isn't a priority in many people's lives—period.

I was recently at the local coffee shop where I ran into a colleague. She was looking distraught. Generally, Carla is a bouncy, smiling, and enthusiastic person, but that day her whole demeanor was downcast. Sitting at the table, slumped in her chair, she barely spoke. I knew why she wasn't herself when she told me that her divorced brother, over fifty years old had just died of a heart attack after a walk in a neighborhood with a friend.

"It was so unexpected!" she relayed and then continued tearfully. "I feel so bad for his kids, because they're going through the house looking for the will and all those important papers to determine what my brother's wishes were, and they can't find anything."

We can't understand how important those pieces of paper can be until death suddenly happens. Lack of planning all too often puts unneeded stress on the family at a time that's already stressful.

As I mentioned before, my parents were organized. They told us, their children, that the best thing they could ever do for us was to make all arrangements for their funeral and have their wills up to date and their personal directives in order. When my parents passed, this proved to be true. When my mom died, the church ladies took care of the baking, the singers knew what songs to sing, and the pastor knew the order of service. My siblings, our father, and I were able to visit before and after Mom's celebration of life at a room in the church. Close friends and relatives could spend time with us, because we knew things were in order and people were taking care of our needs that day. We cherished that time to share memories and food with friends without being inundated with details that needed tending to. Mom had made sure that all was in order.

Crazy as it sounds, many of us don't even have our wills done, let alone any instructions for our loved ones should there be an emergency or life-and-death situation. Yes, I also need to get on that very soon! Life generally works better when we plan ahead of time. When Plan A or B don't work, there are still twenty-four other letters in the alphabet. Putting things into place before life threatens to get complicated is something my parents did in their late sixties and early seventies, when they were relatively healthy, ready to travel more, and of sound mind. My parents visited and met with a funeral director and bought "the package" that takes care of all the details in the event of a death. This was their gift to us.

My mom was the first to pass away. We were so grateful that all the details of her passing had been taken care of, even the cost of the hair stylist for the open casket. And when my dad recently passed away, the same services were rendered. Many funeral homes offer various options to people who want to pre-plan. It's a matter of making an appointment, meeting with the funeral directors, and putting your wishes into place. You have to do the leg work.

My mother always had a grocery list, a to-do list, and even a list of what her funeral would look like, where it would be, who to contact, and what songs she wanted sung. When she was in the hospice at the end of her life, we were somewhat prepared for her passing. When Mom was healthy, she planned ahead so that her transition into aging was less severe. Even though she fought death until the end, her words to me were, "Take care of Dad." What is the plan for that time of life so that transition into aging is not so severe? There are a number of staggering statistics taken from the Vanier Institute that compel us to seriously think about planning for our aging parents or loved ones. Did you know that:

- 28 per cent of Canadians (8.1 million) report having provided care to a family member or friend with a long-term health condition, disability, or aging need recently (2017).

- Most (83 per cent) surveyed caregivers say that their experience was positive, and 95 per cent say they're coping with caregiver responsibilities.

- More than one-third of young carers (36 per cent) arrive to work late, leave early, or take time off due to their caregiving responsibilities, placing Canadian employers at a $5.5 billion loss annually due to caregiving-related absenteeism.

On a positive note, research from Vanier Institute shows that caregiving provides a variety of benefits to caregivers, including a sense of personal growth, increased meaning and purpose, strengthened family relationships, and increased empathy and skill development.

In my case, I was able to be more assertive with the medical staff at the seniors' home and the hospital. I also became quite knowledgeable about a number of topics related to aging, such as dementia, and I passed that information on to my siblings and friends. I also was able to juggle the demands of my life and my family responsibilities and still be an effective caregiver by being more organized.

Eldercare is generally something you can plan for before being thrust into what can be frequent emergency situations. My sister, brother, and I all spent time in different hospital emergency rooms with one of our parents over a three-year period; however, there will always be questions. Scenarios will always arise for which you cannot plan.

The voices of caregivers can be heard around many dinner tables, coffee bars, and hospital waiting rooms. Here are a few caregiver experiences:

I was working full-time when I got the call—Dad had fallen and been rushed to the hospital, leaving mom alone in their home. I "called in the troops" (my brothers and their families) because I wasn't sure if I should head to the hospital or get to Mom as quickly as possible. Someone needed to stay with Mom, and someone needed to be with Dad. We decided who was going where with whom. —Jean

I had recently been laid off work and my wife was a stay at home mom. We'd been trying to make ends meet for the past number of months when we realized that we had to get Mom into a long-term care facility. She only had her meagre pension to live on. Where were we going to get the extra money? Was she going to have to move in with us? —Jeff

I am the only child in my family. Dad passed away peacefully, and I was thankful for that. However, I knew that Mom was not coping well on her own. I felt like I had to step in and take Dad's place. My wife was not in agreement, and it's not working having Mom in our home. I don't want to choose! —Kelly

I work in Toronto. My dad lives in Calgary. I know the laws are different, as are the health care systems. I don't know where to begin looking for help, because I know that Dad needs additional care, and I'm so far away. —Anika

These situations are not unique, but every family has a story and handles their situation differently. In my own family situation, Mom and Dad had done fairly well—driving, living independently, shopping, and travelling ... until about ten months before Mom's death. I remember the morning she called and feebly stated, "I need to go to emergency soon." My panic button was pressed! I was half awake, crawling out of bed and headed to the shower. My heart pounded. I threw on some clothes, grabbed my car keys, and raced down the highway.

My mom's medical situation progressed negatively from that day on, and when she ended up in the hospital for weeks, we realized that Dad couldn't be on his own. As their kids, we took turns moving in to stay with him and adjusted our schedules to accommodate his needs and make sure that Mom had our support and less to worry about. We were inadequately prepared yet we managed. We are a close-knit family and we get along well; however, that's not the case for everyone. We realized that Mom and Dad were getting older, and that we had to start caregiving and taking more notice of what was transpiring.

Our situation was relatively simple compared to the thousands of families who struggle and are not cooperative with each other, or have other issues that are more pressing in their lives at the time. There will always be struggles and other pressing problems, but it's important to put things into perspective. None of us know how long our caregiving will last. It could be days, months, or even years, but despite your circumstances, think of how you would want someone to care for you when you're in their situation in the future. Surrender the anxiety, knowing you're doing your best amidst the struggles. We like the known, the certainties, but life just isn't like that. Encourage one another to get through these times and know that, eventually, life will end—and so will your struggles.

Advanced discussion and planning for the natural life cycle process is essential for families, regardless of race, ethnicity, social position, geographic location, age, or even differences of opinion within a family. Those who do not make plans in advance for the journey of caring for aging loved ones will be faced with frightening and incomprehensible choices at a time that they're highly stressed by the emotional toll of caring for one or more parents or loved ones. Not an easy task.

I recently heard about an agency that received a frantic call from a woman. Her mother was to be discharged from the hospital in twenty-four hours after suffering a broken hip. The woman was desperate for advice. On discharge, her mother was to be placed in a nursing home chosen from a list provided to the family. After a quick visit to some of the homes, the daughter was even more distraught. Only one facility even remotely met the minimal standards she would accept for her mother, and there were no available beds at the time. That's when planning would have been beneficial!

A few weeks before my father's death, he took six ambulance rides in a matter of a few days between the seniors' home to the hospitals. Those journeys could have been prevented had more time been given to transition and better planning. Discussions with the care nurses at the home should have occurred earlier to transition my father. The workers should have explained to me their rationale for having him transported to the city before being admitted to the local short-term care centre in our small town. It was a rash decision based on short staffing and the inability of Dad's facility to meet his needs. I was angry, disappointed, and confused.

So now that you've read about getting organized, having tough conversations, and planning can create ease of transition, you may be wondering a few things:

- Where do I start?

- *I will eventually need to be a caregiver*, might be on your mind, but why plan now?

- If I do plan, how can I make things work in my circumstances?

- Where do I access information about all the things I need to think about, and how will I know if it's even working?

- Are you ready to take that step?

These questions can be answered. That's one of the reasons for writing this book—to aid and assist others in getting answers to caregiving questions. Be prepared to communicate, form your team of support, assess needs that need to be addressed, and make plans. Making a plan is a start. "We can do this!" is a phrase to repeat throughout your journey as a caregiver.

Remember that each province in Canada has its own rules, regulations, resources, and laws concerning eldercare, and the flood of resources, advice, and direction can be overwhelming. Take the information you need and apply it to you as a caregiver and to your loved ones. After walking as a family with my siblings and my parents through this difficult passage, I know how difficult this might seem. This is a guide to direct your journey. Travel safely!

We can do this! I'll say a little prayer for you, and you can make your plan!

CHAPTER 2 TAKEAWAYS:

- ☐ Plan to plan by thinking of the various ways you can get organized in your life.

- ☐ Connect with other caregivers and your support team

- ☐ Assess needs that are concerning you now.

DID YOU KNOW?

Fact: As of November 2018, a non-refundable tax credit may be available to individuals who support a spouse or common-law partner or even a dependant with a mental or physical impairment.

Fact: In Canada, it is estimated that nearly 558,000 full-time employees will be lost from the workforce because of the inability to handle the conflicting demands of work and caregiving. (Vanier Institute)

CHAPTER 3:
LIVING OPTIONS

Concern About the "Where"
Because of Various Needs

"Home is a place you grow up wanting to leave, and grow old wanting to get back to." John Ed Pearce[18]

The first—and last—place most people want to be when they are aging is in their home, feeling what's familiar and comfortable. What are the chances of staying there, remaining independent and feeling secure? Some refer to this stage as "aging in place," but how can we keep seniors in their homes as long as possible? It's not unusual for many of the elderly to remain in their homes until their final breath. But what if that isn't possible? I will cover the various seniors' homes options in Chapter 8.

There are many factors to consider regarding these options, as illustrated by the following three stories. Three stories—three lives— three different outcomes. Trish—Jen— Dany

TRISH'S STORY

Trish's story begins with those casual conversations that go something like this:

Pat: *Bill has been diagnosed with dementia. We're doing okay, though.*

Trish: *Should we start looking for a place that will suit your care needs in the future, Mom? Let's not wait until you're in a crisis. You know how that works!*

Pat: *No, we're doing okay.*

This scenario went on for several years. Pat is Trish's stubborn mom. Bill is Trish's stepfather who had progressive dementia. Trish witnessed his deterioration, but her mom continued to think they were okay. Trish and her sister were worried about Bill still driving. Discussions with Mom got more serious, but they soon discovered that a move to the city would have to happen for both Bill and her mom. Trish made the time to begin exploring available options in the private and public sector.

Bill has since passed away, but Trish's mom continues to live in the seniors' home she moved into four years ago. Trish and her mom approach life one day at a time now, but Trish is thankful that the move was made, and she knows that further conversations with her mom will need to happen.

Just as there are three stories I'm sharing here, there are **three steps** for considering where we or our loved ones want to spend our latter days. We all think about a sunny tropical home on some remote island in an exotic location as we relax and enjoy our retirement years. The travel brochures and financial institutions would have you believe the sunny beaches, perfect smile, and health happen to many individuals. Reality? Ninety per cent of us won't find our way to those beaches.

So what's first?

STEP ONE:

Assess what kind of care you will need in the future. Because everyone's situation is different (living alone, health issues, proximity to family, etc.), educate yourself as a caregiver as to the resources, services, agencies, and assistance available in your area. Look at what supports your loved ones will need now and in the future, whether that's to be able to stay in their home for as long as possible or to move to a more supportive environment. For some families, this won't be an option.

For loved ones staying in their home, there are a multitude of service providers to support just about any need, depending on where you live. This ranges from personal care, housekeeping, and money management to meals and health care. Most of these services come at a cost, though, but some subsidies for personal care services exist, using a specified criteria. A friend of mine was just sharing the option of having a home care worker live in the basement suite her parents have in their home.

Start doing your research by checking websites and government services. Ask individuals who have used these services, as referrals are often the best place to start. Local health care authorities can also provide valuable advice based on the situation. Do your homework by having your loved one's needs assessed by a medical professional. Doctors, health care workers, and family can assist you with determining those needs.

A friend of mine was chuckling about her ninety-two-year-old father, who is still in good health but recently renewed his driver's license and got glasses for the first time! He's still living in his home and is lonely without his wife, who has passed on, but he keeps busy playing pool at the pool hall in town and welcoming multiple visitors to his home.

Keeping people in their homes and communities for as long as possible avoids the costly option of institutional care. It's also favoured by policy makers, health care providers, and many older people themselves, according to the WHO (World Health Organization). They also cite that the number of people over the age of sixty is expected to double by 2050: *"People are living longer lives, so as a society, we need to ensure that those last years are healthy, meaningful and dignified."*[19]

Starting thinking about the topic by asking good questions:

- Is my loved one living alone comfortably?
- Am I concerned about the safety of my loved one?
- Are they having trouble getting around and/or getting to a variety of places because of transportation issues?
- What if more care is needed in the home?
- How much is this all going to cost?
- Are my loved ones bored or feeling isolated?
- What kinds of activities could my loved ones get involved with?
- Would age proofing the home improve mobility and accessibility?
- What are some of the resources they require? Where can I get them?

- What are some concerns my loved ones have about living in their home?

- What can I do to ensure that I am comfortable with having them live alone?

Our family was fortunate that Mom and Dad could remain in their home for as long as they did, but we recognized that they needed some assistance. After we determined what Mom and Dad could afford, we researched various private companies that could offer assistance. All of them were eager to have us "sign up." The agencies gave us a price based on hours. We also had the flexibility to change days and times as needed.

Many of the companies offered the same services at different costs. I made a spreadsheet and chose the top three to share with my siblings and parents. We then "voted" and decided to "try" one for a month at a time. These agencies recognize that care could be for a month or a year, depending on your loved one's needs.

We also discovered that Alberta offers some free care for seniors. You'll need to find what's available in your area and get your loved ones a health care worker based on where they live. Alberta Health Services (AHS)[20] bases their care on assessed need. Their services include home care, supportive living, facility living, palliative and end of life care, and sub-acute and restorative care. Be advised that health services vary from province to province. Do your research. Be practical. Educate yourself. And lastly, take off the Superman-or-woman cape and ask for help or assistance from medical experts or friends.

Mom needed help with bathing, and Dad needed someone (besides Mom) to help him with his compression stockings and mobilize him for his daily walks. They both needed assistance with meals and some light housekeeping. The private company we hired tried to match the workers compatibility to my parents. Mom loved "Mary," but dad was disgruntled with "Nico," who made him walk further than he wanted to go! When Mom, Dad, and I shared our concerns with the agency, changes occurred. More importantly, we wanted Mom and Dad to feel that they were part of the decision making. It also allowed us time to provide and care for our own families. A win-win situation.

We enjoyed some wonderful workers during the time they were employed with Mom and Dad. Those workers shared their lives and expertise with my parents. Our situation included interaction with various workers from AHS and the private company caregivers we employed. It also took the pressure off my siblings and me, knowing that our parents were being cared for when we weren't there. That was not the case with Jen.

JEN'S STORY

Jen's parents had lived most of their lives on their beautiful farm in the country. Her siblings live in their area, and another daughter lives on the property. Jen's parents are adamantly not interested in moving to any facility and won't even entertain the thought of leaving their home, despite the fact that Jen's mom has dementia, and her father is aging rapidly because of worry and care for his wife. He has also been recently diagnosed with cancer.

Because he has taken on the care for his wife, with some assistance from his children, there are concerns about their well-being and safety in their home. I also sense frustration when I speak with Jen about how to convince her parents that it's not in their best interests to be where they are. After her mother had a fall, Jen was concerned that more medical issues would need to be addressed in the future.

The situation continues to worsen, and now her father is in a hospice, her mother in a dementia facility, and the siblings are arguing over what is best for all involved. Since Jen shared that story with me, her father has passed away (in a hospice) and her mother continues to receive care at a seniors' facility.

DANY'S STORY

Dany's story is similar. Dany's mom and dad also lived for years in their home. She and her family lived close to her parents. Dany also has two siblings, but they left all the caregiving decisions to her, the eldest sister. When they had to put their mother into short-term care at the hospital, which ended up being long-term care, the toil on the family was exhausting. Her father still refuses to leave his home for an "institutional facility," even though it would be in all their best interests, as he is now experiencing health concerns himself.

Ask if there are medical complications that need to be addressed. At that point, the hospital or semi-medical facility may be the only option. Perhaps that is the time to start researching various options. Being informed and having some direction is more beneficial than taking the first option available due to urgency of the situation.

A recent study by the Canadian Medical Association found that Canadians are pleased with the health care system's quick response to short-term illness and injury.[21] But the majority of people are not satisfied with the government's ability to provide convenient, affordable, long-term care to seniors. That is disturbing and expensive.

Advance discussion and planning for the natural life cycle process is essential for families. Those who do not make plans in advance for how to care for their parents, or have a plan in place when they need more care, may find themselves faced with frightening and incomprehensible choices at a time when they are highly stressed by the emotional toil of an aging parent. That's not a place anyone wants to be.

My cousins decided that their mother needed more care because she wasn't handling "living on her own" with much success. Their mother didn't want to move and was adamant that she stay where she was. As they were cleaning out her place and packing boxes to give to the Salvation Army, she broke into tears and said, "My life is already full of loss and now you want to throw away my memories? I have loss of health and mobility, loss of family members and friends, and loss of memory and abilities, like forgetting words. Losses. And lastly, I will lose my life soon." She is ninety-six years old and has since moved in with her daughter—with her photo albums and other precious keepsakes. She misses her former life but is adjusting to her new space.

My father, on the other hand, ended up riding in the ambulance to the hospital in the morning for stitches from a fall, back to his retirement home before lunch, to the city hospital in the afternoon, and then transported by ambulance the next day to our rural hospital—getting all the more confused and disoriented each mile of his journey. He mentioned to the paramedics that they needed to check the suspension in their vehicles, as the ride was a little bumpy! We were waiting on a placement for him in a long-term care facility, but he passed away peacefully in the hospital before that ever happened.

A recent article in *Healthy Debate*[22] highlights how preplanned care can mitigate caregiver and patient anxieties, as well as reduce admissions to hospitals or interventions at the end of life. Unfortunately, according to a March 2012 Ipsos-Reid national poll[23], a staggering 86 per cent of Canadians have not even heard of advance care planning! Our advertisers want us to believe that we can use creams and medications to prevent any aging, so why bother discussing it? Most people's health will deteriorate at some point in their later years according to health statistics.

When health problems do begin, it's important to take note—literally—by organizing some sort of medical record keeping. This could mean the difference between staying in the home or being forced to be in the hospital, hospice, or an eldercare home. Therefore, it is time to look at …

STEP TWO:

Keep medical history records and manage the medical care for your loved ones, because it's important to determine if your parents will live in their home or have another one chosen for them when they have medical or health issues.

Because health changes over time and is unique for each situation, focusing on quality of life is important. Get to know your loved one's doctors and health care providers or specialists. These range from podiatrists to clinical psychologists, from orthodontists to gastro-enterologists. Communication with them is pertinent for several reasons. Eventually, you, your loved ones, and supporters will need to discuss various levels of care. These are three:

Comfort Care are interventions directed at maximal comfort, symptom control, and maintenance of quality of life. Attempted cardiopulmonary resuscitation (CPR) will not be tried.

Medical Care interventions are for the usual medical care that is appropriate to treat and control medical conditions. Interventions can be offered. Again, attempted resuscitation will not be tried.

Cardiopulmonary resuscitation (CPR) interventions are for the usual medical care that is appropriate to treat and control various conditions. The consensus is that one may benefit from any treatment, including attempted resuscitation.

Writing down any special instructions that are important for the health care team to know is helpful when preparing goals of care. One can request changes to those goals at any time by simply telling the health care team that further discussions are needed. The health care team will also review goals of care whenever conditions significantly change, which is often the case.

Advance Care Planning and Goals of Care, as well as Health Care Directives are documents that need to be completed. There's currently a movement in Alberta to have all individuals over sixty years of age acquire a Green Sleeve. Just recently, the Green Sleeve has taken precedence over a Personal Directive!

> *"The Green sleeve is a plastic pocket that holds important Advance Care Planning documents and other forms that outline a patient's goals for health care. It is given to patients cared for in AHS who have had discussions, or completed documents, that refer to decision-making about their current or future health care."*[24]

Before Mom went into the hospice, I sat with the palliative care nurse and Mom to complete her Green Sleeve. At Dad's seniors' home, Dad, his case worker, his doctor, and I completed his Goals for Health Care. Be part of those conversations with your loved ones. We experienced wait times in the doctors' offices and engaged in conversations that impacted Dad and Mom's health. I always took my little notebook with me. I remember the day I took Mom to her oncologist. She'd been experiencing more severe pain and was exasperated with caring for Dad and his needs in their home. When she broke down crying in the office, the oncologist gently reassured her that they were doing what they could to help ease the pain. "What else can we do for you?" the oncologist asked.

Mom simply said, "Tell me how much longer I have to live?"

Thankfully and with compassion, her doctor told her, "You have a year."

No one is ever prepared for those words, or for "getting ready to die". Those are stressful conversations, and no one wants to hear those results. Experiencing that moment made me realize that spending quality time with Mom and making sure she was comfortable were priorities for our family.

Mom was in charge of her own health, but over time, she became reliant on many others in the health care system, as well as on family and friends for quality of life before her death. When we finally decided that she needed to go into a hospice, we advocated even more for quality care. Caregiving involves advocacy. There are waiting lists to get onto—not just for nursing homes, retirement communities, and care facilities, but the hospices as well. They are fewer to find and be admitted into. These hospices are available for palliative and near-death patients to have quality of life. Some hospitals are now advocating for a hospice room in the hospital, so that there's more privacy for the patient and the family. The nurses at Mom's hospice informed me that some patients are there for a few weeks, while others are there for longer periods ... even up to a year. When a bed does become available, it's quickly taken. Again, researching, visiting, and inquiring about hospices in your area is enlightening and helpful.

When we knew that Mom could no longer manage at home, her palliative care nurse suggested we start by putting Mom's name on a waiting list. Thankfully, the good Lord saw our need, and we only had to wait a matter of days before she was taken by ambulance to the hospice. We had the option of driving her there ourselves, but opted for the former choice.

I remember the day I took Dad to the hospice to visit Mom. He had his jacket on, and as he pushed the walker into my mom's room, her face skewed, and she motioned for him to leave. When I asked her what was wrong, she waved her arm and said, "the smell."

Thinking that it had something to do with Dad's walker, I took his jacket, got him settled in the armchair in the room, and rolled the walker outside Mom's room.

Later, after I took Dad home, I reached into his pocket and found a bottle of oregano. Mom's sense of smell was very acute, and obviously mine and Dad's were not! I was thankful she had her own room and didn't have the smell lingering there for others as well.

On a more serious note, however, checking out the various nursing homes, hospices, and short or long-term care facilities on the internet or through brochures is beneficial. Visiting them in person is even better, even though it's tough walking those halls and knowing that the people in those beds will not be leaving alive. Imagine that. We can do this, because it was certainly not easy being there.

Getting your loved one's name onto a list, or getting advice from health care providers, ensures that you have somewhere in place for your loved one. Again, there are countless resources listing various hospices and care facilities.

Many hospices only require a donation, because AHS (Alberta Health Services) picks up the cost. Many nursing facilities and seniors' homes require a deposit to hold a placement. In *Passages of*

Caregiving, Gail Sheehy mentions that the conversation with a physician had them discussing values and goals for care at the end of her husband's life: *"Our only regret was that we hadn't had this conversation a year or two before."*[25]

Be proactive and think, with planning in mind. This brings us to the final step in assessing caregiving with our loved ones.

STEP THREE:

Becoming a Quality Care Advocate/Caregiver

Caregiving requires much time, energy, and patience, especially when becoming that medical advocate for aging loved ones. It also requires assessing how they are doing emotionally and where they should be living physically. Being sure that your loved one's interests, fears, safety, care, medical treatment, and access to interesting community activities are addressed are just a few responsibilities of becoming an advocate. I was recently in California and ventured into a convention on Elderly Assisted Living, as I was interested in what Americans had to offer in comparison to Canadian caregiving. Even though my parents had passed away, I recognized that some of my over-fifty friends were experiencing what I'd gone through as a caregiver, and they were unclear about their role with medical staff at the hospital and different facilities. I advised them to be the voice their parents didn't have.

After chatting with a few of the delegates, I became interested in a particular study conducted by ProMatura,[26] a global market research and advisory firm that focuses on levels of satisfaction with services provided and quality of a particular assisted living community to consumers aged fifty years and older. Even though the information was based on an American study, most elderly North Americans fit the description and circumstances. Questions were developed with two goals in mind: focus on sense of belonging and sense of control in their lives. The study revealed the positive "whole person"—emotionally and physically—is impacted by family members providing them (seniors) with choices and the help they needed. Meeting day to day needs and contributing to quality of life for seniors is being met in many elder communities .... at least that's what the research says regarding those communities.

Is that the case in all of them? Not necessarily.

It's the right of every individual regardless of age, ailment, or gender to receive quality medical care and treatment. At times elders aren't able to manage their health care, so as advocates, we must ask questions to ensure their needs are being met. The World Health Organization has much to say about the quality of care for all.

Here are just a few of the many questions every advocate/caregiver should ask should their loved one be moved to a care facility.

- Is the elder respected and treated with dignity, and how will I know?

- Is the doctor or professional taking time to explain and answer questions regarding a health issue or current health event?

- Is the elder offered the best care plan for them at this time and for their prognosis?

- How often is the care plan revisited and revised according to changing needs?

- Are phone calls, emails, or concerns addressed or answered in a timely manner to the elder and advocate?

- Are you aware of all medical issues as a caregiver?

- Is communication between all parties open, understood, and clear?

When a medical history is created, it's easier to prioritize medical concerns and assist the doctor in diagnosis for treating the problem. It should be updated at each doctor appointment. If the elder is unable to verbalize or communicate with the health workers, then it's up to the caregiver or advocate to ensure that the needs of the elder are being addressed. This is why having a case worker for your loved one is important, as they become the advocate for both loved one and caregiver by working out a care plan and filling out the "Green Sleeve." They also have other communication connections that you may not have access to as quickly or readily.

When I'd visit my father in his residential care community, I'd often chat with the caregivers, nurses, and doctors to ensure that I was getting the correct information from my dad. When I was a frequent visitor to the hospital where my dad was a patient, I'd ask questions, inquire how his day was going, and got to know the staff on shift. Being in a smaller facility afforded me that option. This isn't always the case in a larger building; however, social workers and personnel can assist you in any of those facilities.

The positive aspect of advocacy is that even if you don't have the confidence to stand up or voice your concerns, there are generally people in care positions that are able and willing to speak for you. Check at the health information desk at the hospital or doctor's office, or the front desk of senior care homes to voice your concerns. People are compassionate and are willing to help you.

A recent incident that took place in an assisted living centre demonstrates how this gentleman may have had a better experience had he received the correct level of care, even though he had an advocate working for him.

Residents who lived at this centre enjoyed apartment style accommodation and ate at a central cafeteria. One morning one of the residents didn't show up for breakfast, so a table mate went upstairs and knocked on his door to see if everything was OK. She could hear him through the door, and he said that he was running late and would be down shortly, so she went back to the dining area.

An hour later he still hadn't arrived, so she went back up toward his room, and she found him in the stairwell. He was coming down the stairs but was having a bad time. He had a death grip on the handrail and seemed to have trouble getting his legs to work right. She told him she was going to call an ambulance, but he told her "no," he wasn't in any pain and just wanted to have his breakfast. So she helped him the rest of the way down the stairs and he had his breakfast.

When he tried to return to his room, he was completely unable to get up even the first step, so the health workers called an ambulance for him. A couple hours later, a call was made to the hospital to see how he was doing. The receptionist there said he was fine. He just had both of his legs in one leg of his boxer shorts and they were driving him back home![27]

Part of this gentleman's care plan should have included dressing assistance in the morning and at night. This was a humorous incident, but it can be frustrating to those vying for assistance for their loved ones. If your loved one refuses medical help or treatment, as was the case with my friend Jen's parents, it's probably best to develop and try various tactics to get them the help they need. Some of these might include:

- Having a doctor make a house call (if you can find one who will do this).

- Finding a better or different doctor if there's an unresolved issue. Don't be afraid to ask for a second opinion. It's your right.

- Suggesting a visit to the optometrist, dentist, or physiotherapist.

- Visiting a less-threatening medical environment, like a walk-in clinic.

- Attending all appointments as the advocate/caregiver to ensure nothing is missed, and to act as a second set of ears for those with failing hearing.

The key to ensuring that your loved one is comfortable with the medical attention they receive is to use compassion and positive "sell" tactics to convince them that seeking medical help, or having daily help, is in their best interests. Let them know that you are worried about them.

"Dad, I noticed that you seem really tired and aren't very energetic recently. Can we just check with the doctor to see if you're as healthy as you can be? I won't worry as much when we find out what's going on."

Taking those "preventative" measures, such as visiting a doctor, before things get serious is something to consider. You are the caregiver/advocate, but as much as possible, let the elder(s) you're concerned about being part of the decision making, and help them keep their dignity. Because people want to be in control of their own lives, we have to be sensitive to taking over and controlling our loved one's life. Being a caregiver/advocate is not about control; it's about compassion.

Elder-care Canada[28] is an advice and action consulting service business based out of Toronto, but they are available to anyone in Canada as well as internationally. There are multiple resources to assist anyone who needs more information on issues ranging from increased health challenges to support services for each of the provinces.

Being proactive, talking about topics such as additional assistance needs or illness, and planning for our loved one's future seems unpleasant at the time, especially when there are no major concerns to address at that moment; however, it is critically important. When my dad had one too many falls when he was living independently, choices were made for him as his family, care workers, and the staff at the retirement home were fearful for his safety. A variety of fears could surface in the future. Sometimes it's not even about health issues.

Many elders fear that they'll run out of money and be financially unable to live comfortably in the future. There are also as many who don't want to burden others with themselves and any health problems that go with them. Older adults, often ones who have lost a loved one, are lonely or feel they have no purpose in life, especially if they have few hobbies or interests. Some fear neglect or abuse, moving from the family home, or memory loss or dementia. Add medical issues to those fears, and stress increases for all parties involved.

Being proactive and advocating for a better future doesn't require any specific skill set beyond what most of us have already. Don't be afraid to reach out to someone you know who has gone through the journey. Many adults are parents or caregivers, so when it comes time to have meaningful conversations, we already have experience under our belts.

The best skills you can bring to the process are the abilities to listen, ask questions, have compassion, and develop resourcefulness. After having gone through the past few years as caregiver and advocate for my parents, I'm now able to encourage and offer advice to my friends and colleagues who are on this journey themselves. We can do this! You can help someone plan the next steps on his or her journey, whether they're living alone or in a medical assisted facility.

For example, my neighbour is a self-sufficient, energetic eighty-seven-year-old woman who still drives, goes for her daily walks to the mailbox, and enjoys friendly conversations with those of us along the block. My father, on the other hand, was an aging, passive, non-walker who needed care. Everyone does need to be heard, respected, and cared for in some capacity. Some just need more advocating than others.

When the phone rang at 4:30 in the morning months ago, my sister-in-law, who had been visiting from out of town, wondered who one earth was calling at that hour of the morning. She and I headed over to my dad's seniors' home. Apparently, the situation was dire. They could not locate my father.

"He's not in his room, and we can't phone the police because he's living independently. We know he's in the building, because his safety wristband tells us. We've looked everywhere."

One hour later. We jiggled door handles. We looked outside with our cell phone flashlights. We checked cupboards, the games room, nooks, and crannies. The door with no name—unlocked by one of the workers—was the last option.

There was dad. My heart cried. He looked so helpless standing naked in the empty room, telling me that he couldn't get out of the huge building he was in. He had locked himself into an empty suite on his floor after wandering from his room that night. When the workers went to check on him, he hadn't been in his room.

After this incident, I was concerned and immediately advocated for more care by speaking to the staff. I asked that changes be made to the system that was in place and requested that they move my dad to the memory section of the home with the support of the staff, my siblings, and his case worker. None of that came to pass, but I was in contact and communicating with the transition nurse and case worker to ensure that Dad was taken care of in his independent living space, because it was beyond what I imagined could have happened. We're not always in control of what happens, but we've all invested time, interest, and energy into our loved ones and the elderly. They are worth our efforts.

Because of my dad's situation, I was reminded that we all work better together. Allow the lines of communication to stay open. When we "partner" with our loved ones or parents, rather than impose our opinions and decisions without their consent, the relationship is healthier, and parents or loved ones are more open to discussing issues and hearing our perspective. But if they can't comprehend those decisions, then we have to make choices in the best interests of all involved.

When we work together for the benefit of the individual—namely, your loved one—we use our gifts. I'm always amazed at how generally patient, caring, and firm the nurses are who work with dementia patients, and I often felt "bad" that I couldn't help my dad out more than I did. I remember one occasion when Dad was in his last weeks of life at the hospital. I'd gone for a visit, and he was adamant that he was going to "bust out of the place" and get himself some cigarettes. They had to strap him down into his wheelchair because he was literally trying to get up out of the chair and out of his room. I found it difficult to see him "chained" to the chair, but I knew that the nurses did this for his safety, as they couldn't sit with him 24/7. I really felt helpless, because he was in no condition to be walking at all. I would have loved to "bust him outta there," but not to go buy cigarettes!

My sister put things into perspective when she said that these are professionals trained to work with these individuals. It's part of their job, much like many people probably felt "bad" for me teaching all those middle school kids in my teaching career. We all work together for the best interests of those we care about. In my case, as a teacher, it was the student, other teachers, and the parents I cared about. Then I retired and it was Dad, the care workers, such as nurses and doctors, and our family—who worked together for Dad's best interests. I was thankful for all of them.

Because of the care needed, individualized for each situation, the greatest benefit to all parties is communication. Their voices and our voices need to be heard, but when we can keep smiling despite our present situations, we know that we're simply doing our best for the ones we love.

"*Wrinkles should merely indicate where the smiles have been.*" Mark Twain[29]

CHAPTER 3 TAKEAWAYS:

- ☐ Think about and **assess what kind of care you will need** in the future. *Based on my health concerns at the moment, what kind of care will I need?*

- ☐ **Keep medical history records and manage the medical care in partnership with the elder(s) and medical professionals.** *Do I have a folder with all the medical records?*

☐ Be sure that your loved one's **interests, fears, treatment, and explanations of medical jargon** are understood by being an **advocate** for them. *Have I assured my loved one that they are being cared for in the best possible place and the best possible way? And if they are not, am I willing and able to speak for them?*

DID YOU KNOW?

Fact: Hospice is for anyone facing a life-limiting illness, regardless of age.

Fact: The majority (more than 60 percent) of hospice patients are diagnosed with conditions other than cancer.

Fact: Hospice is not only a place; it is a service that can be provided wherever the patient may be—in their own home or a family member's home, a nursing home, or an assisted living facility. Hospice is also provided in inpatient units, veteran hospitals, and some correctional facilities.

CHAPTER 4:
COMMUNICATION

Building the Team for Emotional Support and Connections

"Kind words can be short and easy to speak, but their echoes are truly endless." Mother Theresa[30]

The best time for having a discussion about pre-planning for eldercare is **now.** Even if your loved ones aren't mentally competent, having an effective plan requires initial communication with siblings, caregivers, and all involved in your loved one's life at the moment. Make sure that an official document, like a Power of Attorney, names the representative who can speak for your elders. This doesn't need to be complicated, even if there are many members in the family. Being an only child doesn't always mean that all the responsibility is given to that person, either. The representative can be a family member or a trusted friend.

There are a variety of methods of communication; face to face or voice to voice are effective for some people, while emails helped me convey information, feelings, and thoughts to my siblings. I'm a journal writer, and expressing things in written form gave me time to express what I needed to say.

Be clear what it is you want to communicate.

A recent story I read in a magazine in a doctor's office illustrates the importance of effective communication.

> Apparently one day, a new nurses' assistant came into a hospital room. She found a man sitting there fully dressed in the chair by the bed. There was an overnight bag by his side and it looked like he was ready to go. She showed him the wheelchair, but he was adamant he could walk by himself without any aid. Wanting to follow hospital procedures, the assistant was insistent that rules were rules and so he relented and got into the wheelchair and allowed her to push him out to the hall to the elevator.
>
> As they were descending, she asked him if his wife was coming to meet him at the front desk of the hospital.
>
> He replied, "I don't think so. It takes her awhile to change her clothes, so she's probably still upstairs in the bathroom taking off her hospital gown and getting dressed. She'll wonder where I went."[31] She was the patient getting discharged!

When communication is effective, everyone gets the same message. On one occasion, I was to take Dad to a doctor's appointment, only to find out that his doctor was on paternity leave. The case worker at his seniors' home told me it would be two weeks until his return, but the receptionist at the clinic informed me that it was actually two months! I was a bit miffed and wondered what confusion that could create when the doctor's office and the health workers weren't in sync.

Sharing information and getting answers to questions is helpful. At times you'll feel that the lines of communication have been torn down, or that no one is "getting back to you" in a timely manner.

Hang in there and keep calling. Keep talking and discussing. Your persistence will pay off, and they will get to know you. Remember that thought about advocacy? You are your loved one's voice when they can't speak and need to be heard.

Because having proactive discussions when seniors are in good health is more beneficial to all involved, it's important for one person to take that first step to ensure that there even is a discussion. It could even strengthen family ties and encourage thoughtful communication with all parties involved, namely the elderly and caregivers. I tend to communicate through phone calls, text messages, and emails. I tried to make personal contact when possible, and as our parents' needs arose or continued to develop, I assessed the situation and made sure everyone was informed. Our family often shared ideas, and we discussed issues and came to a consensus—whatever was in the best interests of our loved ones.

We should even start thinking and talking about our own plan to put into place! Alberta Health Services is proposing mandatory plans for all people at age sixty-five, to ensure individuals address issues before end of life. This project is in progress.

By deciding who is going to take the lead, the family could avoid a potential emergency. Ongoing communication will also help maintain the emotional stability of the whole family in the crisis, should there be one. I would send monthly or timely emails or make phone calls to my siblings to keep them up to date as to what was transpiring in my dad's life, health-wise and mentally. My siblings were thankful for this, as they weren't there day to day. They did have a number of chuckles, which is evident in this particular email:

Good Morning to All! (and a beautiful one at that!)

Just a quick update on the last few days/weeks with dad.

Tim and I had a chuckle yesterday, as Tim came out to see dad in the morning for a quick visit. When Tim got home, they called him and said that dad was downstairs waiting for him to take him fishing. They told dad not to leave the building and he said, "Tim is always on time and has just gone to get bait." Nonetheless, I arrive later to take him to his Doctor Appointment (get ears cleaned for his Connect Hearing test next week to fix his hearing aid that he hardly wears!) and he is sitting in his chair with hat on and a sweater on his bed. I ask him, "ready?" and he asks, "Where's Tim? We're going fishing." I say where? and he says "up in the mountains"—that's why he had the sweater. He continued to mention the fishing all afternoon. I say to him, "Where's your fishing rod?" I don't know he says, "I think I gave it away to one of the boys."

The night before he called myself and Tim and said that he was having trouble breathing when he lays down. Tim and I both told him to push the green button! He did, J, the health worker came and settled him in for the night. When I asked him about it yesterday, he said, "I just take a bunch of really deep breaths and go back to sleep." They are also trying to get him to drink more water. He told me they made him drink 6 glasses at once yesterday. When I speak with the gals, they just say that they are happy if he drinks a glass.

Nonetheless, we have all noticed a gradual decline in the memory and a bit of confusion. I explained this to Dr. K yesterday and we will get a Chest Xray, CT Scan asap for his Hydrocephalus (one year ago he got one).

We went for his Specialist appointment with Dr. B and he sees that the meds that dad is on for the "Blow outs" is working - so we will continue to monitor that and he won't have to have the Intravenous drug. His blood work looks normal from last time as well, but we will get that done every 4 months. He still has Crohn's but loves his bacon!

Some of the other little things that I am noticing (and I am sure there are countless others...)

When we were at B's office, he went into the washroom, came out with no walker.

He came down to the nurse's station as I was coming in - said that he got mixed up on the wrong floor and came down to get oriented.

He called me and told me the new housekeeper's name is Lori. How did I spell my name because he wanted to see if it was spelled the same way.

He asked if he could borrow my computer to do a presentation on horses. He loves the book you got him, Peg and wants to drive to Saskatchewan to get the next version and visit his parent's gravesite.

Yet - other times, he is sharp and remembers lots of stories about his childhood. He spent about half an hour yesterday telling me about Uncle Laurel and the wild horses. He also remembered Susan's husband's name when I showed him a picture. He also gets irritated that G calls him every week. I told him that she loves and cares about him.

Anyhow—we will continue to do what we can. They have a new manager coming for the Senior home this week, so hopefully things will work out for the guy as the staff is carrying the weight of running the place without a leader. BTW - I took in some flowers and a card and thanked the staff for all their hard work and running the place without a manager. They are appreciated and little R, D and lovely J are certainly helping dad stay on the Independent side for as long as possible. Dad's AHC case worker will continue to assess dad's condition and I will need to touch base with her soon.

I am off to the city for my hearing aid adjustment and a hair cut. Tim and I hope to take dad for an ice cream and a ride on Saturday. He enjoys the weekly outings (supper last Saturday) and weekly phone calls or visits.

Love to all and let's enjoy that beautiful, sunny weather! ☺

We know that: Psalm 121:8 *The Lord will watch over your coming and going both now and forevermore.*

Everyone has his or her own style of communication, and that was just mine! Individuals in families have their own connections. You will find yours.

In my family's case, I was deemed in charge when there was a crisis. Because I'm the eldest and recently retired (semi), I was responsible for getting things started. I was also delegated to the role of executrix for my parent's will. Each of my siblings also took on various roles as the needs of my parents arose, but someone had to get things moving. This isn't always the case, as there may be dissension in the family or only one child—or perhaps the family isn't close, either geographically or emotionally. At times there may not be a family member wanting to take on the role, so ensuring that there is a close family friend or other relative available is essential to make those connections.

Being sensitive to how we go about communicating is also something to take into consideration. Even though there will be breakdowns and barriers to communication, it's important to show empathy as a caregiver to all involved. That way, Mom isn't left in the hospital room without a wheelchair, and Dad can be at her bedside waiting for her! Hopefully, family members will see the positives of your role as communicator.

There are always exceptions to every circumstance, such as: single children with no one to help them with the decision making; the parent of a child with special needs who needs to make time for both parents and child; or the caregiver with health problems of his or her own.

So, you are the "chosen one" to take the communications lead. Where do you start? There are basically four things that may be helpful: recruit your team of supporters, gather resources and information that will guide you, maintain a positive outlook, and share your loved one's story and legacy.

First of all, before any conversation can take place, it's important to get all the facts and start compiling a list of resources that you might need to convince your loved ones that something needs to change. This is when you start to notice those little red flags that things might be changing in your loved one's life.

Having medical information from health care professionals is essential to differentiate the facts from the fears. For example, Dad wasn't allowed to take certain medications with other meds. He also had to have his meds at a certain time in the day, so when we'd go out for lunch or leave the building, we needed that information. By attending appointments with your loved ones, you can discern what is going on and not have to rely on your parents' memory. You are informed. Then let your family members know the facts as you learn them. Keep them "in the loop."

Accepting the fact that loved ones are aging and aren't as independent as they were in the past is important. Some elderly people don't like being reliant on others, and making any adjustments in their lives is a struggle. Help them to see that you're not a threat and that they won't be losing their independence either. Have your advocates understand this as well.

Because aging is a complex matrix of issues, one must be sensitive to your loved one's concerns, history, and decision-making. The need for respect must be in the forefront of any of those discussions. To ensure that the trust is there, lots of questions need to be addressed. Simply giving advice isn't good enough. Sometimes listening and understanding where they are "coming from" helps. Many studies indicate that having a sense of control is pertinent in seniors' lives. After all, how do we react when our "power" is taken away from us?

I distinctly remember experiencing that feeling when I was teaching a Grade 8 Language Arts class. One particular boy in class would often challenge me and get some of his classmates riled up and into heated discussions. The vice principal happened to be walking by the class and stuck her head in the open door, observing the student making his point quite emphatically.

"Out in the hall!" was the command. Many students, including this young male, were startled and started to ask, "Why?" She then began to name other students and had them sent out as well, and then down to the main office. I will never forget that feeling of power loss and not being able to say anything at the moment, because she was the authority figure. I was humiliated in front of my students. Don't make your parent feel that way. We can change those feelings by working with dignity, respect, and love.

Some helpful ideas to try could include exploring different possibilities with them, offering choices, and validating feelings to give your loved ones a voice in any of your discussions. Make them feel a part of what's happening. For example, when we decided that Dad needed to be in a retirement community because we knew that Mom's time was short, we discussed how he felt about living on his own, even though Mom was still alive at the time. This put Dad at ease, because he was part of the process in choosing a site in which to live. We also looked at the possibility of Dad living closer to my brothers in the city, but he wanted to be in a smaller community. We often had to chuckle, because he loved the smell of the "barnyard," and his room ended up overlooking the rodeo grounds at the edge of town!

Time, love, and laughter can bridge some of the disconnects and offer a smoother road to conversations. We can never assume that we know what's going on in our loved one's minds. We also don't know what they're feeling unless we ask them. It's our job to ask valid and personal questions to get honest answers. Because elder issues are also family issues, it's important to hear suggestions and ideas from all members, regardless if you're the one in charge or not. When you look at the common goal and what's best for everyone, it helps to see the bigger picture. One wants to be caring and loving, not overbearing, insensitive, and manipulative. Yet at certain times I suppose I was insensitive to Dad's requests. He would often want to come over to my place, go out for supper, or have me eat with his table at the seniors' home. I'd tell him that I was busy or that it wasn't a good time, when all I really wanted was a break from the weekly routine.

One wants to be an effective communicator. So, what are some of those great communication skills and questions one could ask oneself?

Let's try asking some of these:

- Am I being sensitive to what my loved ones are feeling and saying?

- Am I listening intentionally without being biased?

- Am I being fair and open-minded to everyone's ideas in the family, even if I don't agree?

- Am I struggling with some of my thinking and own issues and feeling resentful?

- Am I making assumptions and maybe need to review the facts?

- Am I showing empathy toward others?

- Am I helping my loved ones with solutions to their/ our problems?

- Am I initiating and following through with conversations?

- Do I need more information to make an informed decision?

- Am I asking the right questions?

- Is this a family issue that needs more resources or time to discuss?

- Are we taking things step by step?

- Is there a trust issue with anyone?

- Are we avoiding decisions based on lack of information?

- Do we have all the facts?

There will always be doubts and decisions that need to be made; some decisions will be addressed periodically, while we will need more time with others to come to the right choice about what is best for our loved ones.

One of the healthiest ways of adding life to years is simply positive thinking. We can foster that with our loved ones by communicating positively. There will be all sorts of personalities involved as well, so it's often best to take the "sunny side" or the "cup half full" attitude. Humour also helps when dealing with stressful situations. One can create humour by simply not taking everything so seriously, even though there may be times when screaming would be the other option.

If family members have disputes, it's best to be that advocate and try to resolve any issues. Seniors, like anyone, find it stressful to hear loved ones fighting; however, someone needs to be in charge. Just as families are unique and diverse, the same can be said about seniors!

People age differently—just go to a mall, visit a park, or head to a nursing home. You'll see older adults with walkers, many sitting docile for hours or being anti-social, while others exercise in a fitness class, go for daily walks, and drive. Some watch their diets or welcome new challenges or positive opportunities, while others are adverse to any change. The world has much to offer, so how can we renew, rejuvenate, and inspire more positive elder quality of life? Because there's no social system in place to maintain or reinforce quality of life, it's up to the family working cooperatively to acknowledge and carry on the values, traditions, culture, and memories of our loved ones. Hopefully they will share with us their stories and inspire us to look ahead to our futures.

Secondly, because we want to stay positive, we have to face the fact that our roles as caregivers have to be positive. Change is inevitable and constant. Despite the fact that we may see our loved ones' lives deteriorating, or they may be struggling with health issues or negative attitudes, we need to remain caring, "upbeat," and approachable about a variety of topics, issues, and circumstances. Trust me—at times I put on the "positive attitude" when all I felt like doing was staying home in the bathroom, crying, so no one could see the chinks in my armour. I needed to vent and release those feelings of frustration. At other times I'd phone a few friends and go for a coffee. I also had a group of Christian women who stayed with me after church to talk, and we met weekly for a Bible study where most of our time was spent talking about how stressful life was. There were always my sisters' morning inspirational messages and nightly phone calls. Most importantly, I prayed, sang, and journaled.

Recently, a friend shared that she never cried, had headaches, or felt overwhelmed, but that all changed when her mom took a turn for the worst and she had to spend overnights assisting with her mom's health concerns and becoming that advocate in her family. She needed "backup," encouragement, and positive influential thinking. Thankfully, she too has a group of friends who talk with her, give her advice, and pray for her. Her brother also moved closer to their mom to help with the responsibilities and care, so her workload lessened.

Not only do we need to be alert to the signs that our loved ones may need more care and are less independent, but we also need to "share the care." Relying on communication between a network of family members and friends, community volunteers, and health care practitioners is mandatory! This worked well for my family because we were sharing texts, emails, and phone calls on a regular basis. We also had Mom and Dad's friends, who would visit and give encouragement to all of us. Finally, I developed a professional relationship with Mom's and Dad's doctors by talking with them privately and going to all of my parents' appointments.

Our parents were very independent. My mom drove to all of her and Dad's appointments. They would house sit for friends and family on the west coast during the winter. They would visit all of us siblings and our families in various locations. They were generally happy and able to handle their finances, even though the odd time they would forget to send a birthday card. Then Dad had his first fall.

Taking time to address Mom and Dad's concerns and our growing worries about them gave us the opportunity to find out what was on their minds. When we communicated with them about some of their issues, they were willing to discuss them, which allowed us to start sourcing out a team to address those needs. We were fortunate that we had that connection. Some families don't have that bond, so it's important for your loved ones to convey their concerns to someone they trust.

We started by making a list of things Mom and Dad could still do, things they needed help with, and things they refused help with. We looked at all of our schedules and availability and came up with a sketched-out plan to start. Again, we were fortunate to have a larger family. If that's not possible, then you have to build your team with volunteers, other friends, and groups. Get the community to assist you. It's about teamwork.

My sister-in-law and I could drive them to appointments during the day. My brothers could help with buying the groceries, visiting and checking up on them, or taking them out to dinner or an outing on the weekends. We had to coordinate my sisters' out of town visits with other family and friends' potential "help times." We literally had a desktop calendar posted on their fridge for easy reference for all of us (including Mom and Dad) to see how the "care was shared." Recently, a friend of mine said that they used that strategy as well to keep track of all the appointments, who was helping on a particular day, and the names of the care workers coming in to assist her parents. That's where we were.

Initially the level of care was minimal, but as Mom's cancer continued to ravage her body, and Dad's dementia started to cause more concerns, we needed to add members to our team. Added to our list was a group of volunteers from my parents' church. Mom and Dad also had friends from the neighbourhood who helped out with meals, but we eventually had to rely on affordable, professional care providers. That's when we started researching the potential care providers in the area. We soon discovered that there's a wide range of caregiver services, from co-workers and friends or siblings to government agencies, support groups, and health care providers. Some at a cost. Once we had the list, we had to establish how each of the individuals and groups could help.

We also reviewed a budget to determined what our parents could afford. We found numerous agencies on the internet that provide a variety of services. You need to hone in on your loved one's needs and wishes. Service availability also depends on the area you live in. Even hiring someone to come and live in the home, or having your parents live with you, are options. Every situation is unique and should be carefully considered.

Thankfully, my parents lived in Alberta, which has a health care system called Alberta Health Services (AHS). At present, they are the forerunners in providing numerous and various services to all Albertans. Their website is easy to navigate and provides a wealth of information on various topics surrounding physical and mental health. There are countless resources within the Calgary area to assist in determining where to start.

Unfortunately, though, caregiving tasks can't always be equally distributed among family members. Because my sisters lived in other cities, my brothers had work commitments, and we had limited finances, the primary responsibility remained with me. This is often the case when taking on the role of caregiver.

According to the Canadian Medical Association (CMA), caregivers are the backbone of society. Statistics show that 5.4 million Canadians are providing care to a senior family member or friend.

This care was most often received by a senior in their own residence; the most intense care provided by those living with the recipient. In all, 62%

of caregivers said the care recipients lived in a home separate from theirs, while 16% were living with the recipient and 14% said they provided care to a senior in a care facility. The Statistics Canada study found that 56% of caregivers living with the recipient provided at least 10 hours of care a week.[32]

As well, there is little coordination between provinces when it comes to financial support for family caregivers. Manitoba has legislation recognizing the role of caregivers, and Nova Scotia provides assistance for family caregivers in lower income brackets. Some financial supports are in place at the federal level. Many individuals juggle caregiving with their employment, which causes a strain on their family. Recently, the CMA has called on the federal government to make changes to the Caregiver and Family Caregiver Tax Credits to make them refundable. This would increase financial support for family caregivers.

Improved communication between the provinces and the federal government would benefit individuals involved in this "business." Things are changing as advocates speak out.

I remember the day that I went to check on my parents and found out that my then eighty-five-year-old dad had been helping lift my eighty-year-old mom into and out of bed in the morning and often several times in the night. Dad was getting very interrupted sleep. But the "straw that broke the camel's back" occurred when I asked Mom how she was managing to get up from the toilet seat. She informed me that she was pulling herself up using the towel rail on the wall by pulling the towel. That's when I knew much more care was needed. There was no discussion on that particular topic!

We started asking the four basic questions to get more supports:

- What kind of help was needed?

- How much was this all going to cost?

- Which agency had the best care or kind of help we needed?

- What programs could complement or supplement the kind of home care needed for our parents at this time?

I set out to research. I developed a chart to find reliable, competent, low-cost in-home helpers. I also asked other individuals for recommendations, and I had a list of questions from my sister that needed answering. All this information was helpful. We then narrowed our choices down to three agencies based on our needs. There are many helpful resources on the internet. For example, www.elderindustry.com has a geriatric list for case managers to assist individuals wanting resources. The first option is always trying to keep your parents or loved ones in their own home.

After communicating with my siblings, we made our choice and clarified expectations, reviewed the contracts, and modified our agreement based on my parents' needs. Now we were prepared to set the plan into action, but there was always the question: "What's next?" Did we have the right care we needed for our parents? We thought so at the time.

Now that those options were clarified, we realized that our parents' cord of life was slowly coming unravelled. Time with them was now more important. This is not the case in some families, but fortunately for us, it was.

More families and "teams" need to create as many positive caregiving moments as they can. There are a variety of ways to do this, but do it before it's too late. Organize life celebrations, spend quality time together and make memories with aging loved ones. We can impact the lives of younger generations and create opportunities for elders to feel valued and give back to the family.

We decided as a family that we needed to share the joy of having Mom for yet another month, so shortly before she passed away, we invited friends and family to her eightieth birthday. We created a poster board with photos so that when people arrived, they could write a message on a stickie note and post it on the board. We wanted to list the eighty reasons we loved Mom. She read them later with tears in her eyes. We also had a mini talent show with lip syncs choreographed and acted by the daughters and nieces. My sister made a box of eighty chocolates—that Mom loved! My niece and brother performed a rendition of Forrest Gump and the famous "box of chocolates" scene. My favourite line was *"Mama always said life was like a box of chocolates. You never know what you're gonna get."* The best part, though, was the fact that Mom watched all of this in her wheelchair, with her sisters on each side. The smile on her face as we sang "Happy Birthday" and celebrated being there together with her family, including her great-grandchildren, will never be erased from our memories.

Lastly, what's a better way to communicate love and care than to make memories, share "living lives," and have elders communicate so that you have their legacy to share when they're gone?

My father loved genealogy. He used to spend countless hours researching, connecting with relatives, and compiling that information into huge photo albums containing stories, photos, and family trees. My eldest son and nephew hope to continue that research. They used to spend time listening to my dad's stories. My hope is to one day compile his stories into a book he started to share with his grandchildren and my siblings.

Find those boxes of photos, awards and trophies, home movies, newspaper clippings, artwork, and mementos, and listen to the memories and stories that go with them. You can also scan photos, put them on the TV screen, and watch and talk about them. Everyone can get copies digitally as well.

Planning engaging conversations and keeping and sharing family traditions, customs, and rituals gives an opportunity to bind the family together. The most treasured gift we can give is our time, so prepare to spend quality time with aging parents or loved ones when you can. This way, both the caregivers and the cared for are able to share experiences and connectedness. I know that Dad often looked forward to the "next event," whether that was a visit from a family member or friend, a supper at my house, or a birthday party. I truly believe it sustained him for as long as it did after my mom passed away. Your loved one's health will determine what activities you can embark upon. You can, however, do some simple things.

Some ideas for consideration, depending on availability, location, and cost, might include:

- taking a class together to learn something new

- going through old letters, photos, or memorabilia and having those conversations about what those items mean

- venturing off to community events such as teas, theatre, choral group singing

- watching old videos or films

- writing a note, letter, or card to family members

- creating a family bulletin board with photos

- throwing a celebration of life party!

- treating them to a restaurant or outing in the park, or even inviting them for dinner

- checking their "bucket list" and choosing another item to accomplish

- attending a sporting event by buying pregame tickets
- staying in touch weekly with emails or phone calls
- sending a care package
- redecorating the living space
- inviting youth or grandkids to read to them
- giving them patience and a listening ear
- countless other ideas
- Be creative!

Many positive aspects of sharing and communicating with loved ones can evolve from simply planning to spend time together. This can afford opportunities for laughter, fun, and personal love and bonding. It can also open the door for more serious conversations.

My girlfriend shared that her father seemed to be slipping into a bit of depression because he loved woodworking, but his eyesight was failing and he was having difficulty seeing. When they finally got him into the shop and had some people assisting him, he was able to get back to what he loved.

I got into the habit of taking my dad for a Sunday afternoon drive. Sometimes it was just a drive through McDonald's for an ice cream cone to eat in the park. Other times we took a drive in the country to sit on a bench overlooking the mountains.

Once in awhile we visited a local landmark or small business to check it out. There are countless videos, stories, and memory ideas on various sites across the internet, but make your own memories to keep and share with others.

I also sat with Dad when his mind was a little clearer and we wrote his "story"—the accomplishments, memories, and moments he remembered from his life that mattered. Like the time he and Mom were met with a shotgun and a lady behind it telling them to "get off her land" when they went to explore an old barn in a field. He loved working with barnwood, creating picture frames, bookcases, and a variety of items. He and mom were always on the lookout for old barns to stock his pile of materials—thus his connection to the old barn and the old woman! Luckily, they weren't arrested for trespassing, nor did they need a good lawyer to fight any charges.

Speaking of legalities and good lawyers … that's the subject of the next chapter.

CHAPTER 4 TAKEAWAYS:

- ☐ Start compiling not only a **list of resources** but a team of supporters that you can communicate and share information with. *Do I have your group of supporters?*

- ☐ Our role as caregivers has to be **positive.** *Do I have a positive outlook on life that I convey to those I love?*

- ☐ Have elders **communicate so that you have their legacy to share** when they're gone. *How am I getting my loved ones to share their story?*

DID YOU KNOW?

Fact: The topic of end-of-life is on people's minds. Three-quarters of Canadians (74 per cent) report having thought about end-of-life.

Fact: When asked, most people indicate that they would prefer to die at home in the presence of loved ones, yet almost 70 per cent of Canadian deaths occur in a hospital. (2006)

Fact: When asked about the importance of discussing end-of-life care with different types of individuals, six in ten Canadians surveyed (61 per cent) say that having the discussion is extremely important with at least one individual. (2006), yet only 13 per cent have an advance care plan prepared.[33]

CHAPTER 5:
THE LAW OFFICE
All the Legalities and Paperwork

"By the time you're eighty years old you've learned everything. You only have to remember it!" George Burns (1869-1996)[34]

There are numerous issues to address before a death, let alone what happens after a loved one passes on, just as there are numerous lawyers, accountants, financial planners, and other professionals who have a variety of experiences, qualifications, and services to offer for a fee. There are also differing laws across the provinces if a person passes on with or without a will. Even the legal jargon can be confusing at times. It's sometimes a challenge to navigate all the legalities and their purposes.

In layman's terms, there are basically **three** important documents to have in place when planning. Seeking legal advice and ensuring these documents are legally valid makes it easier for caregivers to provide care, often results in less cost and time compared to alternative court applications, and enables your wishes to be followed. After all, pre-planning is about making things less complicated for loved ones and caregivers.

1. **The Will**—This document lets the individual decide what happens to property, personal items, and monies after death. You decide who may administer your estate, handle your funeral arrangements, and follow your will.

   There are various types of wills. They can range from a formal, typed will completed at a lawyer's office to a will entirely in one's handwriting without witnesses. There's even the case of a Saskatchewan farmer who used his pocket knife to scratch his will into the tractor's fender.

   Things to include in the will can be found on numerous websites; however, a lawyer can simplify and guide you through the process based on your particular family situation and assets. Be careful of the pitfalls of doing it yourself, as a lawyer will ensure you consider your legal obligations to others. For example, if you are married or common-law, have minor children, or disabled adult children, a lawyer can assess whether the ownership of your assets aligns with your will. A lawyer will also determine whether your assets' designated beneficiaries align with your will. Failing to properly address such issues when drafting your will may result in your will being overturned by a court, or your assets being distributed contrary to your wishes. Depending on the complexity of your situation, a lawyer may consult your accountant and/or financial planner to ensure the will aligns with any tax and/or financial plans. Be sure to read the drafts of the documents carefully, as lawyers or their staff can make errors, such as misspelling a name.

2. **Power of Attorney** (General and Enduring)—This document lets an individual choose someone to make financial and property decisions if the individual is incapable. It's important to note that the individual making the document—the

"donor"—needs to be of sound mind for the document to be legally valid. The difference between General and Enduring Power of Attorney is that the Enduring Power still has effect after one loses their mental capacity. When my brother and I were at the lawyer's office with our father, we were asked to leave the office so that the lawyer could speak with dad privately. The lawyer had to ensure that the donor was not unduly influenced by other people, as someone may later claim that the document was legally invalid for that reason. Proper pre-planning allows those decisions to be made beforehand to avoid complications later on when your loved one may not be in good health or of sound mind. **Also know that Power of Attorney is only effective if the donor is alive.** A lawyer can assist you with properly preparing the Power of Attorney.

3. **Personal Directive**—This document enables an individual (the "maker") to choose someone to make medical and other personal decisions not concerning finances and property if they are unable to or incapable of doing so. These instructions only operate while a person is living. They can be as detailed as one wants, but the Personal Directive is often intended to cover the maker's broad wishes.

A lawyer can assist you with properly preparing the Personal Directive to address broad medical and personal decisions.

Some makers who live alone, or who want their appointed agent in the Personal Directive to have more specific direction about the maker's wishes, beliefs, and values, will choose to have a Green Sleeve that works in conjunction with the broad Personal Directive. You should not rely solely on the Green Sleeve, as the Personal Directive covers personal decisions beyond only medical decisions in the Green Sleeve. Do-it-yourself Personal Directive forms are found online and they differ from province to province. One does need to consider the pitfalls of not obtaining legal advice and having the documents properly executed and commissioned. You may spend less money having your lawyer prepare the Personal Directive and other documents from the beginning of the process instead of doing them yourself without legal advice or asking for legal advice after doing the documents yourself. Either way, you are completing the process, and that's what matters!

Recently, another colleague of mine relayed a story of heartbreak as she explained that her brother decided to take over her father's affairs. She and her sister trusted that their brother would do everything in the interests of their father, who was living out of province and near him. This was not the case. After her father's passing, they discovered that their brother had liquidated all estate assets and cleaned out their father's accounts and investments. Because nothing was in writing from their father, the brother felt he had no obligation to his sisters. The girls were devastated, and are no longer on speaking terms with their sibling. Because the father did not have a will, the Provincial Will legislation will likely dictate who will share the father's estate. The brother may even be liable to repay those beneficiaries. Not all stories are fairy tale endings, but justice does sometimes get served.

UK statistics indicate that over 26 million people have left no formal instructions for what should happen in the event of their death. But what about in Canada? A recent BMO report on estate planning found that 48 per cent of survey respondents did not have a will (2017). As well, another survey discovered that at least 12 per cent of people with wills had out-of-date documents.[35] Where do you stand?

Also note that you must ask permission to use a person as your executor. They have the right to decline. Not everyone wants that role, as it can be very time consuming, onerous, and frustrating if not all papers are in order.

Choosing the right person for the role is something to take into consideration when you do get a will. Because laws change and decisions need to be updated, it's important to know that everyone, regardless of age or wealth, needs a will. They are serious business and they won't cost a fortune to have prepared.

Lawyers can provide high quality services. They are extremely knowledgeable and helpful and were patient with our aging father. They can simplify matters for each unique situation, administering estates properly and addressing all the legal issues pertaining to those circumstances.

There are countless resources on the internet, as well as self-help books, if you're seeking information about legalities.

Now that you have the documents, it's important to let your appointed attorney(ies), agent(s), and executor(s) know where those documents are placed, hidden, or filed. These people could be your trusted family and friends. If you use a lawyer, he or she may store the documents at his/her firm in a safe and provide photocopies for your reference. Your appointed attorney(ies), agent(s), and executor(s) would then only need to contact your lawyer for assistance in activating the Power of Attorney and Personal Directive if necessary during your lifetime, or in administering your estate after your passing. That would simplify things and one wouldn't be searching for the documents when they're needed.

Original documents do need to be kept in a safe place. As a caregiver, be prepared to show those documents to doctors, nursing home managers, or other key people. Also be prepared to deal with doctors, a lawyer, and financial and other institutions as the Power of Attorney and Personal Directive may need to be activated with forms between the doctor and the appointed attorney(ies) and agent(s). The lawyer will then need to prepare notarial copies of the documents for delivery to the financial and other institutions. All those papers again! Even though completing all this may seem overwhelming, these forms need to be completed so that your job will be easier later on.

My parents had a large portable file folder. These are often sold at stationery stores like Staples. They stored their important papers and documents in it for easy access. After my sister organized the various paperwork, it was an easy task to locate certain papers when Mom went into the hospice and then later passed away. I also used it to keep all the important papers for my father. It was also very handy when income tax time rolled around and when we needed proof of Dad's income and Mom's death certificate!

Mom had indicated in her will a cost for hairdressing. We found it a bit odd, thinking that she had requested a closed casket. Knowing Mom, we knew that she wanted to look her best, even on her death-bed. After careful review of documents prepared, in the event of her death, we discovered that she had requested an open casket and, yes, she included the hairdressing cost to ensure she looked beautiful, which she did. God rest her soul.

Caregivers may often find valuable information that was not relayed to them by their parents or loved ones, and may discover these facts in organized files and legal paperwork. There may be some surprises and frustrations, like my sister's friend experienced. Carla had to go through copious numbers of drawers, cupboards, and closets to find the property taxes on her dad's house, his will, and a variety of other papers scattered throughout his home after he passed on. It took considerable time and effort, but after almost two years, some of the legalities are finally getting sorted out!

Meanwhile, costs have been incurred from her bank account to take care of "tidying ends up." A costly cleanup to say the least that could have been prevented. Just as there are numerous unique situations, each family deals with their circumstances in all sorts of methods and means; however, the law does prevail.

There are also countless legal terms that individuals need to understand when dealing with the law. However, retaining a lawyer should reduce the need for you to understand countless legal terms, or at least explain many of them. I remember wondering what on earth *probate* was. Originally, I thought it was a payment to the government on the money that we inherited from our parent's estate. I did find out that probate is the legal process in which a will is reviewed to determine whether it's valid and authentic. My dad's banker had us hire a company to take care of the general administering of Dad's will, but they also dealt with estates where there was none. The company explained the process, and they had their own lawyers to go to court and take care of the estate details at a fraction of the cost of just having a lawyer and doing it ourselves. The secretary I dealt with was very patient when I inundated her with emails full of questions regarding the legal process.

As mentioned previously, the will is a crucial document because this is how an individual wants his or her estate "divided up" when they pass on. The executor or executrix's job is to carry out the directions and provisions stated in the will. In my case, my brother and I were co-executors, but after Dad passed away, we realized that it was in our best interests to have just myself—with more time and availability to meet with the lawyers and sign the various documents. In many cases, it can be a friend or even one family member who is entrusted as the executor. Sometimes having more than one executor can create problems, especially if one is out of province or country. Having an executor who is out of province may also create tax issues for the estate.

Sometimes people may benefit from creating trusts during their lifetimes in combination with a will. An example of this would be a person who has a blended family and/or significant assets. A lawyer who focuses on these specific trusts can assist. You may also create a trust in your will for a spouse, children, disabled adult children, and others. Again, being of sound mind and body and having these conversations well before a situation arises that needs to be dealt with can be beneficial to all parties. My father's financial advisor shared a few horror stories with us about elders who were coerced and manipulated into giving up large amounts of real estate and investments. That open communication is of utmost importance!

Because the executor's job can be demanding and difficult, not to mention that it leaves one open to family criticism and risks of personal liability, recognition of the value of services can be received, and the executor is entitled to compensation. If the amount is substantial, it can be used as taxable income. Any fee is taxable, substantial or not. A way to counter this is to set out in the will that the executor is entitled to a specified bequest in lieu of compensation. When this is done in advance, it may preserve family harmony, and the monies will go to the chosen beneficiary instead of some of the alternative executor's fee going to the government as income tax.

The problem with this is that a specific bequest may be insufficient for the executor's efforts, the size of the estate, and the time to administer the estate. Trying to avoid taxes by setting a specific dollar gift amount may result in inadequate or excessive compensation. Some people choose to leave it up to the law, which enables the executor to seek the residuary beneficiaries' approval for a fee. It would likely be taxable income for the executor. Other people choose to set the percentage, but it may ultimately be unfair. My lawyer suggested the 3 per cent rule on moderate estate settlements, which simply means that a reasonable fee should be collected due to the time, commitment, and effort it takes to complete the process in the role of executor.

Because I'm the executrix—now called "Personal Representative"—of my father's estate, I could write an entire book on the duties, pitfalls, and legalities of that role. Needless to say, there are several books on executor role and duties. In Alberta, the Estate Administration Act (available online by googling Alberta Queen's Printer) also has a convenient and brief schedule detailing the core tasks of an executor. As well, through some financial institutions, a person can contract companies to assist executors and provide services for a fee.

Another document that can be useful is the Letter of Instruction. This doesn't require a seal from a notary or lawyer, but is simply a letter to guide the closing affairs of a person after death, as well as a list of people to notify, explanations for the funeral arrangements, or any other personal details that need attending to after death. *This is not be confused with the will, which is a legal document.*

Just as there are countless costs, resources, and legalities to address, there are also financial matters to resolve. These often go hand in hand with some of the legalities.

Probate is a word many of us have heard but rarely understand. It's basically the process of validating the will and the executor as confirmed by a court of law. There are three basic techniques to avoid probate costs or at least reduce them.

First of all, joint ownership allows the right of survivorship. With the death of the first joint owner, the survivor automatically becomes the full owner of the assets, subject to any legal claims. In some cases, however, the capital gains and income tax are more expensive than the probate costs saved. One has to be careful when considering adding an adult child or anyone else as a joint owner, as that may restrict your ability to sell such assets during your lifetime. It will also give the joint owner full access to the assets, and it may be contested after your death and result in an expensive legal battle if the surviving joint owner did not contribute his/her own money to your joint assets.

Another technique to avoid probate costs is the designation of beneficiaries where legally permissible. Legally designated beneficiaries will receive assets such as RRSPs, RIFs, TFSAs or life insurance policy monies more quickly and any debts outstanding cannot be touched by creditors of the estate, as such assets do not form part of the estate.

Lastly, trusts created during one's lifetime separate from one's will— also called inter vivos trusts—are instruments that hold assets and remain in control of the trustee during his or her lifetime, according to the terms of the trust and for the benefit of the beneficiaries. Depending on the terms of the trust, the trust assets pass to the named beneficiaries without probate. Again, capital gains taxes may have to be considered. Trusts are complex, and lawyers and accountants should be involved.

Your best bet is to hire a reputable lawyer and have paperwork completed, kept up to date, and filed away in safekeeping for the day you will need it.

CHAPTER 5 TAKEAWAYS:

☐ **Do I have all the legal documents in order?** *Double check I have the documents.*

☐ **Do we have a reputable lawyer?** *A responsible lawyer ready to explain. One can be found by word of mouth, friends, co-workers' suggestions, bankers, or reading reviews on line.*

☐ **Do I understand all the legal terminology and jargon?** *Lawyers can simplify complex vocabulary. Can't afford a lawyer? Call the* Legal Aid **Alberta** Legal Services Centre at 1-866-845-3425 *and they will give you advice.*

DID YOU KNOW?

Fact: Current demographic data shows that the percentage of Canadians over sixty-five is increasing rapidly. This increase is often expressed by the term "greying of Canada." Frustratingly, to date we do not have sufficient information and research to provide a clear picture of the hurdles that Canadian elders face in accessing justice.[36]

Fact: Senior women outnumber senior men in Canada.

Fact: The ability of an older person to communicate effectively about their legal needs is another common hurdle to justice. Lawyers are trained to address the needs of various demographics and take care when addressing issues that can arise when assisting elderly clients with their estate planning documents (mental capacity, undue influence from others, communication issues).

Fact: Likewise, elderly sub-population groups (LGBTQ+ elders, senior females, social, cultural, religious, and ethnic minority elders) struggle with their unique socio-cultural barriers to accessing justice.

CHAPTER 6:
THE BANK—FINANCIAL
MATTERS

What about the Money?

"The great thing about getting older is that you don't lose all the other ages you've been." Madeleine L'Engle [37]

Again, the best time is **now** for initiating and discussing issues and topics regarding money and future financial plans. When we consider the best interest of all parties involved in conversations about money, it's more effective when we look at all the finances that are affecting or will affect our parents.

Reviewing your loved one's finances is important for several reasons.

First of all, family members may be in for a surprise, one way or another, about how little or how much is in their parents' bank accounts, not to mention their investments. According to the Bank of Canada, the oldest unclaimed balance in a bank dates back to 1900. When a Canadian-dollar account has been inactive for ten years, and the owner can't be contacted, the balance is considered unclaimed. Unclaimed monies are transferred to the Bank of Canada once a year on December 31st. Approximately 2 million accounts, worth $816 million, were unclaimed at the end of 2018.[38] On the other hand, if information had been made available to a trusted individual, many of these accounts would have been claimed.

Because many caregivers think the federal government or provincial health care will cover many of the costs of aging, they may be in for yet another surprise when they go to research long-term care or nursing homes. The harsh truth is that it costs money to live a long life. Changing needs of loved ones will dictate how much money is needed for our lifetimes. When we pre-plan at an early stage in our lives, we know we need to have money for our basic living needs, health expenses that emerge as we age, and our lifestyle and growth for the future to be able to do the things we'd love to do when we're older. We also need money for investments or leaving our legacies.

My husband and I decided that we would pay off our mortgage by the time our sons had finished high school. That way, we could continue using the money to pay for their university education. Thinking ahead afforded us the ability to fund their degrees, but how many individuals even factor in cost of living increases or anticipate what it will cost to live in a retirement home or hire someone to assist when living at home? I know that my mother was determined that both her and dad could live comfortably in a seniors' home until they were well into their nineties. Unfortunately, neither lived that long, but she had suggested that she had six children for a reason—to help her and dad when they got older!

Most financial planning includes three types of opportunities:

Non-controllable are things like struggling with health issues, suffering a serious illness, becoming dependent, or dying prematurely. Many people have life insurance for this reason. **Controllable** are things like debt-reduction, personal savings for retirement or education, and even a home or investment property. One can pour as much money as they want into any of these to reduce debt or invest.

Growth opportunities occur when a person is preserving the estate or maximizing his or her wealth. If a person has his or her finances in order, money can be invested.

There are countless advisors who give financial advice and want to ensure that your money is used to aid and assist you into older age, rather than hinder and cause caregivers to deal with debt later on. Check any financial institution or insurance company and they can provide that assistance and information to help you make informed choices. Choosing a financial advisor is important business.

Unpaid caregivers who are taking care of family or friends are in a different position than professional caregivers who provide a paid service; however, the financial stability of the elder is important for the unpaid caregiver to know, because if there are expenses incurred, they need to be paid. At times, financial sacrifices may need to be made for various reasons. Some caregivers reduce their hours or give up their jobs to support or care for their loved ones. There may be a mix of formal and personal, or informal, care provided. Paying for some sort of service while the caregiver remains employed and juggles the responsibility of a caregiving role is an option. When care is no longer possible in a home, then the caregiver must be on a full-time schedule, and that can be expensive. The caregiver might need to give up their employment, or hire someone to care for their loved one full-time. When individuals can anticipate the need for adequate long-term care, then many issues and problems can be addressed beforehand and certain steps put into place.

Even something simple like knowing the average cost per month for a room in a nursing home is helpful, as is working on a budget to predict costs in the future. Having those conversations with loved ones helps establish those predetermined costs for a later time.

My parents were frugal and had savings and investments. They sat together with my brother and I, who were deemed executors of their will. They projected the cost of living should they reach a certain age, what the costs would be if they continued renting after selling their home, and how long they could afford to live in a seniors' or dementia facility should their life come to that. I remember the scene well. Dad always kept meticulous records of his credits and debits to the last penny. I remember Mom even buying pantyhose with the groceries so it didn't look like an added expense. Nonetheless, we got the paper and calculator on the table and tallied up possible scenarios. We had a list of the potential homes that could accommodate Mom and Dad's needs and then added up the numbers. We narrowed their choices down to three places and then went and visited them to reaffirm their decisions and get more information. Some of their friends mentioned to my parents that the price you pay when you move in will not be the same from year to year.

Understanding these options in advance results in more satisfactory experiences; handling a crisis saves money and opens the door to other options because prior research has been done and decisions made. Because care is complicated and varied, expensive and uncertain, caregivers and loved ones need to have these pre-planned discussions earlier rather than later in life—even though it may be uncomfortable. It's important to review your elder's current finances. Then there are less surprises and conflict over who is covering what costs.

According to a 2012 BMO survey,[39] seven out of ten caregivers were providing some sort of financial assistance to their aging parents or relatives. In Alberta and British Columbia, local health agencies will assess your loved one's needs and their ability to afford care. Based on these needs and how much help is available, the province offers so many free hours a week of support.

The government of Canada also offers Senior Assistance for lower income individuals. One must apply for this; however, the paperwork is worth the time invested. Shar's ex- husband had been off work for a number of years due to health concerns. He was living in a rental apartment and barely making ends meet. She agreed to help him out by filling out the paperwork required to prove he was in a lower-income bracket. The government subsidized his rent and afforded him time to get to all his medical appointments. Thankfully, we live in a province that assists people.

Even though there are subsidized retirement home rates for seniors, they are in high demand and often have long waiting lists. Other options include no government funding and using private funds to subsidize government pensions to pay for housing and care. Regardless, paying for eldercare requires planning and preparation, because the cost of hiring privately also works out to $20–$80 per hour for more personal care.[40]

My parents sold their house and then invested their money. My mom was able to budget carefully to calculate how many years they were going to be able to afford living off their investments. She also calculated their Old Age Security and Canadian Pensions. The average senior will have up to eighteen years of good health and ten years of bad health, according to the statistics. My mom, thankfully, didn't have to suffer ten years of bad health! When she passed on, Dad became a single pensioner. Luckily, his income was minimal and he received some government assistance, which he had to apply for—rather, I, his caregiver, filled out the proper forms and submitted them.

Any individual sixty-five years or older can calculate their income to see if they qualify for the Seniors Financial Assistance programs through the federal government. Now that Dad has passed on, his estate is entitled to death benefits from the government; something Dad collected when Mom passed away.

Another tidbit to note is that as of 2011, an individual is allowed to give someone up to $13,000 a year without having to file a gift tax return. As well, if you provide more than 50 per cent of the financial support for a loved one, or anyone for that matter, you can count those persons as dependents on your income tax return, as long as their income is under $37,000 a year. Medical expenses can also be claimed as deductions on your return. Be sure to save all the receipts from any prescriptions and medical bills to use when you file your income tax.[41]

If your loved one cannot pay for basic accommodations, subsidies are available based on tax returns and depending on which province you live in. Friends of mine recently moved their mother from Ontario out to Alberta. There are certain laws pertaining to health care wait times and transitions for each province before health care "kicks in." Each province has its own laws and regulations governing these topics. You'll need to research the laws, as they are continually changing as governments and health care changes.

As many cases as there are for positive pre-planning, many families mismanage the funds from the elderly and seniors. Some of these elders don't want to report financial abuse, so troubles are left in place. Some possible red flags that caregivers, trusted friends, or siblings and relatives can watch for might be things like:

- suspected misuse of Power of Attorney
- changes in bank account activity or investments noticed on bank statements

- pressure to sell or remortgage the home

- opening a joint account with an older person who is not a trusted friend or member of the family

- physical or verbal abuse from family members or other caregivers

Nonetheless, planning financial strategies do work well for both caregivers and ones who need the care. Having peace of mind because you have a properly prepared plan in place is thoughtful and beneficial. Expressing concerns regarding our elder's ability to remain financially stable in the long run helps all of us when we prepare to do the same. Because when the money runs out, the family or caregivers typically pick up the costs of care. Do you want to be financially responsible or strapped in your older age? What might one do to prevent that from happening?

When seniors find it difficult to keep track of money, it's time to visit the bank. Ensuring that the Power of Attorney is able to write cheques or have access to the debit card for accounts will hopefully see family members happy that someone is taking care of the finances. We can do this by being transparent with the funds.

Start with a budget worksheet. The first question to ask is: What is your loved one's total income or assets? **Secondly**, what are their average monthly expenses? List everything from medical, food, and housing to travel, housekeeping, and long-term care insurance. If you're working with a financial advisor, choose one who will discuss and analyze long-term eldercare finances with an understanding of longevity. Be sure to review insurance policies and look for senior discounts such as elder programs and Medicare (Blue Cross), bus passes, or even community services.

CPP (Canadian Pension Plan) and Old Age Security from the government is available to seniors, but there are also programs and assistance for people living on limited incomes. Check those out on the provincial and federal government websites to see if your loved ones are eligible.

One factor that some people may not have considered is how to manage money from another province or country for their loved ones. Perhaps establishing an online bank account is the best option in this case. Having a trusted friend or family member manage finances for you is also an option. Another point to consider is if there are pensions from other countries. It's best to check those details so there are no surprises.

When my mom, who had taken over the finances from my father for years, finally succumbed to her cancer, someone needed to ensure that the estate was settled, bills and rent were paid, any outstanding balances and accounts were up to date, and the managing of funds for Dad were in place. We had gone to appointments at my parents' financial institutes prior to my mother's passing, so that when the transition to take over the accounts began, much of the paperwork, the probate, and other documents were signed and in place.

Because many of my dad's expenses were simply automatic payments each month, we ventured out once a month when he needed an outing and a little cash from the ATM. I "assisted him" in acquiring funds, and we knew that we would need to take over all of his financial interests. I was honest and careful regarding my father's expenses as his financial manager, but I know that some families have different stories to tell about individuals depleting their loved one's accounts and causing major rifts in families. Not all families agree on financial decisions. These were the least of my worries; however, my dad did call me at home one day from his retirement home quite distraught.

"There's a bill here for $23,000!"

I told him I would come over and have a look at what was going on and offer an explanation for this distress. After reviewing the paper he'd handed me, I realized it was his rental receipt from the facility in which he was living. I was so thankful I was handling his financial affairs! Numbers can be confusing for the elderly, so someone needs to explain information to them in a coherent manner so they're not distraught or worried.

I also took the various receipts and invoices and filed Dad's papers in a file storage binder for safekeeping. I also informed my brother of where it was and what it contained. Now I just need to get my affairs in order and go through papers in my desk, drawers, and safe and let my sons know where all the documents and important papers are before I forget where I put them all! Which brings me to my health. After countless visits to the banks, setting up appointments with financial advisors, and then explaining it all to Dad later, not to mention keeping my own finances in order, I was ready for a treatment at the spa!

CHAPTER 6 TAKEAWAYS:

- ☐ **Start** with a budget worksheet. *Have I got the numbers correct?*

- ☐ Estimate the **average monthly expenses.** *Have I estimated correctly?*

- ☐ Work with a financial adviser, who will **discuss and analyze long-term eldercare finances.** *Who is my adviser? Are you meeting regularly about once or twice a year to address your assets and finances?*

DID YOU KNOW?

Fact: 20 per cent of Canadians are still working past the age of sixty, while 56 per cent of Canadians sixty and older face at least one form of debt.[42]

Fact: Financial abuse is the commonest form of abuse against the elderly and will often go unreported. This includes manipulation or exploitation of someone else's money, using elder's money or property dishonestly, and failing to use their money for the older adult's welfare.[43]

CHAPTER 7:
THE WELLNESS SPACE

Physically—Mentally—Emotionally—Spiritually

"There's no such thing as aging, but maturing and knowledge.
It's beautiful, I call it beauty." Celine Dion[44]

We've all heard the saying, "Take care of yourself or you can't take care of others." My sister often paraphrases the airline attendants' speech with: "Put on your own oxygen mask before you assist others." But the question remains: How do you care for yourself when there are so many demands in the role of caregiver? Because of the many demands on you as a caregiver, you can be stretched in a thousand directions, and your health seems to be the last of the list of "to do's."

My siblings have been kind when offering me advice about some of the caregiving decisions, but friends of mine have had critical opinions thrown their way. I have, at times, resented the fact that I needed to give up a day to take my dad for an appointment, or spend my afternoon sitting with him when the conversation was revolving around what we talked about three days in a row. It was certainly not my dad's fault for where he was, and I'm grateful for the time I did get to spend with my aging parents.

Sometimes I had to sacrifice a work day, a coffee with a friend, or a trip to the city because I needed to be around for my parents. That's part of the role of caregiver—being there when our loved ones need us. This can cause friction between spouses and family members because of the time commitment, so communication is pertinent!

The time I've had to take off work to be sure that all the paperwork and caregiving was attended to is minor when I know that giving of my time benefitted my dad. Thankfully, I have a faith and am a firm believer in balancing my life. For me, balance involves three areas that can get "out of sync" at times. However, knowing what these areas are and how they work for me, I can readjust, gain perspective, and return life to a manageable state. Properly managing these areas positively impacts our well-being and overall health. We can do this! You can plan to manage your life! I also say a little prayer for me.

Physical—the health, exercise, and "out and about" demands

Mental/Emotional—the mindset, fear, frustrations, emotional roller coaster ride

Spiritual—connecting through prayer, meditation, music, writing, and time for "me"

So when my dad had a "blowout," I, the staff at his seniors' home, or my brother would clean up the mess. Dad had Crohn's, and when nature called and there was no washroom to get to quickly; the mess ended up in his Depends. Sounds so undignified. It was messy. Dad invented the word "blow out" as our family term to indicate when he would have an accident. I ended up keeping an extra Depends in my vehicle, and my brother and I visited many a men's washroom to help Dad clean up. Mom had also suffered embarrassment from Dad's accidents at airports, in the grocery store, or when they had company for supper. The laundry was a daily chore.

Like Mom, I had to tell myself it was part of Dad's condition and say a little prayer of thanks if his "blow outs" happened close to home. On other nights Dad would call to say that he couldn't get the TV channel he wanted. I'd tell him to check his menu on the TV and locate the correct channel.

"Take the channel changer," I'd say. "Put in the numbers 1–5–9."

Then I'd hear the *beep, beep, beep* in my ear on the phone.

"Not on the phone, Dad. Punch the numbers into the channel changer."

"Oh, that's way over on my chair. It's too far away and the numbers here are bigger and I can see them."

I know that he needed to hoist himself out of the kitchen chair, take his walker to maneuvre three feet over to his Laz-Y-Boy, and find the channel changer. I told him not to worry. I'd ride my bike over to his place and be there in about ten minutes. That way I could say a little prayer, get some exercise, and know that I'd helped him out so he wouldn't be frustrated for the rest of the evening. Fortunately, I didn't live too far away. The weather was generally sunny and the bike trails were clear!

Friends have stories of parents calling and asking them to fix the internet or adjust the TV channels, not to mention trying to locate certain items they have misplaced. The trouble is, they're miles and sometimes provinces away from their loved ones. That's when they rely on others to care for their parent and hope and pray that it's sufficient.

The demands on caregivers are great, and stress plays a major factor in the decisions that need to be made. If a caregiver isn't careful, his or her physical health can come into jeopardy. Too much work, not enough sleep, and eating improperly are just a few of the reasons stress occurs. I remember rushing back and forth from my house out of town to my parent's place, to the hospital and hospice, and grabbing a burger to chow down on from one errand to the next. I should have kept more water and a few healthy snacks in my vehicle. I do now, but back then I just didn't think it that important … until I got irritable.

There are various signs to take note of when caregivers aren't doing well.

Symptoms can include feelings of hopelessness (I'm at the end of my rope; I'm anxious that not everything will be taken care of). Then there are the tears and sadness, or not taking part in things once enjoyed, simply because of lack of energy, time, or effort. Getting angry, losing concentration, not sleeping, feeling tired all the time, and losing or gaining weight because of dietary changes are also signs. Increased drinking and smoking, along with increased health problems, can also be a concern and aggravated by little exercise, excess tiredness, and overall stress levels. There are many variations of stress, and they manifest in each of us differently. Health is important. I have IBS, so I know that stress can come in many forms and manifest itself in many ways.

"Taking care of a relative or friend has its own set of stressors that can disrupt sleep. Recent research shows that 76 percent of caregivers report poor sleep quality-and female caregivers, who outnumber their male counterparts two to one, are more likely to be among them. One reason: Female caregivers may spend as much as 50 percent more time providing care than male caregivers do, and researchers think there may be a threshold of time beyond which the likelihood of health consequences-including poor sleep-escalates. And regardless of gender, 'being a caregiver is tough

on your mental health,' says Dr. Sharkey. 'If your loved one is ill or has dementia, you may become sad and anxious, which affects sleep.'" [45]

When you can honestly attest to the fact that you think you're not doing a good job as a caregiver, or when you start feeling guilty about not saying "yes" to your loved one's requests all the time, or you simply wonder if you should be doing more, that's when you need to safeguard your health and take action. That "vice grip" is now a death grip on your health and needs to be loosened.

It's been proven that long-term stress can lead to serious health problems, so it's important to get "moving" to help take care of or alleviate the added stress of being a caregiver.

How do you manage the physical balance, and what are some activities to ensure you stay in good physical health? Many people have a routine exercise program, go to the gym or workout somewhere by doing something to boost their physical health. Because caregiving can consume your time, it's important to schedule those exercises to keep physically healthy in one form or another. It also boosts the immune system, improves sleep, and, yes, energizes you!

These exercises could be as simple as a quick walk, bike ride, or yoga YouTube video on the computer or iPad. The recommended time for exercise of any form is at least thirty to forty minutes, three times a week. If that's not possible, then even little "bursts" here and there work as well. After all, ten minutes is better than no minutes. Park your vehicle at the edge of the mall parking lot and walk briskly down the aisles of the supermarket or store. Take the stairs. Challenge yourself to "keep in shape." I use my exercise bike in my basement, turn up my music, and pedal. I also pick up my girlfriend and head to Aquafit once a week, even though it's offered many times. Walk with a friend. Walk alone. Walk. Get doing something, though.

To ensure your health is in order, be sure to visit your own doctor if you have any health concerns whatsoever. You'd be surprised how many people forfeit their health by brushing aside health concerns and pay for it later. Not something you want to put off doing.

Getting adequate sleep, drinking enough water, and having a good belly laugh are also beneficial to your health. Connect with a friend who makes you laugh. Head to a comedy at the theatre, or watch a humorous TV show. Fill that water bottle up and even set a bedtime and the alarm for waking up to establish a routine.

It's also easy to neglect your eating habits, so a good tip is to ensure that you're eating healthy and recognize when you're hungry or feeling low on energy. Fresh fruit and vegetables are important, so keeping healthy snacks around is nutritious for you and your family. Getting outside every day also boosts the spirits and increases Vitamin D levels, weather permitting. This is a vitamin we lack, especially in the winter (at least here in Alberta).

Just because you're a caregiver, don't deprive yourself of the time and care you need. If you don't take time to look after your own physical health, you won't be much help to your loved ones. As a bonus, if you can get your loved one involved in the physical exercise and care, then it's beneficial to all!

Ideas for fun and getting physical include:

- Go for a walk around the block, down the hall, or around the building or to the mall—just get up and walk.

- Dance—disco, waltz, aerobics, chicken dance.

- Fly a Kite—head to a park and enjoy being outdoors, even if it isn't windy!

- Take the dog for a walk—or let the dog walk you.

- Go to the fitness or exercise room and lift weights or get on the exercise machines.

- Visit www.passportforwellness.com and exercise in your chair while travelling the world.

- Attend a local yoga class or try one online.

- Participate in a charity walk.

- Stretch.

- Bike around town or on bike paths.

- Hike—it's good for the soul.

- Swim or join an Aqua class.

- Join a seniors' sports league.

- Play Wii or board games with the kids and grandparents.

- Splash in the waterpark or run through the sprinkler.

- Shovel the neighbour's walk or mow their lawn.

- Rake leaves and then jump in them.

- Head to a health food store and ask about superfoods or elixirs.

- Ask a friend or others for ideas.

- Explore hundreds of websites for activities.

Now that you're up and moving, how do you stay *emotionally and mentally* positive as a caregiver? There are countless self-help books and websites that give tips on caregiving, but three top items that continually show up are: *taking care of yourself, talking about what you're going through, and staying positive!*

Because we can't control much of what's happening with our aging parents, it's a fabulous idea to maintain that positive mindset with a conscious effort each day. By filtering the negatives from our lives—such as not watching the news for hours on end, not listening to people who bring us down, or preventing things that drain us emotionally—we work at developing a positive mindset. Mindfulness and thinking those positive thoughts require rewiring our brain.

A variety of resources and tools exist to assist the caregiver in managing negativity or stress. Check any wellness caregiving site and you'll be inundated with a variety of helpful information.

First of all, think practicality! By prioritizing and breaking tasks into smaller jobs, things become more manageable. Delegation of duties is also beneficial. For example, I liked to use my Tuesdays, which was the day my dad's housekeeper cleaned his room at the seniors' home, for volunteering, doing my dad's laundry, paying the bills, and even having a cup of coffee with a friend. By connecting with others, you're able to talk about your stress. Some people even join support groups to provide that encouragement for the caregiver.

I was also thankful that I had close friends, dear sisters and brothers, and a church group that helped me with different tasks and understood what I was going through. I had conversations with them, and they were able to encourage and support me with words, hugs, and empathy.

These meaningful relationships and friendships can last a lifetime, and the social network of support is crucial for emotional connectedness and well-being. When you're unclear or unsure about what's happening, talk to an expert in counselling to help you through this transition in your life, especially if there's no one close to confide in. Many workplaces provide benefits packages that include psychological care.

Recently a friend of mine said that she'd been to a support group, but when she asked where they went for coffee after the information meetings, the senior organizer said, "Oh, we don't have those anymore, because all everyone did was complain!" The point of a support group is to encourage and help each other out, because everyone is going through similar circumstances. After she told me about this, I offered to be her support person, and we now meet for coffee every few weeks so that she can vent and share what's working and what's bothering her about caring for her dad. Find someone that can just listen when you need to share.

By accepting help, you also relieve yourself of unneeded stress. My good friend and colleague would often pop in to visit my dad. She'd drop off goodies and provide a cheery disposition to my parents when my mom was alive. She'd been looking to volunteer, as she had recently retired. She knew them and had started seeing a decline in her own mother's health, so she understood to a certain extent how time consuming and emotionally draining caregiving can be. She is such an adoring, beautiful woman with so much compassion! She is on my Top 10 list!

It's easy to make a list of people and their interests. You'd be surprised at how many people are often more than happy to help you out when they see the need to relieve you and give you a little break. Having those groups of volunteers and network of people is important. Again, check what groups are available for your support network. And more often than not, we can give back what others have offered us when they go through their "journey."

Getting connected with other caregivers and learning all you can about caregiving resources in the community where your loved ones reside, gives you a better picture of the landscape in which your loved one lives. Learn all you can about your parents' health diagnoses and focus on what you're able to contribute to their care. Even find out about your medical leave if need be. Nearly 60 per cent of caregivers are employed, so if stress levels are rising, take time off the paid job for a while to alleviate some of that stress. Many workplaces also have plans, and bosses are often sympathetic to workers' situations.

Because we're often so independent, don't have time, and struggle with asking for help—let alone wondering where to get assistance—it's important to take advantage of any assistance we receive. Isolation or depression can leave a person struggling on their own. That is not where you want to be!

Tim Drake shares ideas to help with emotional or mental health in his book, *You Can Be as Young as You Think.* He suggests that the most important thing in keeping young "is a positive mental attitude being the absolute essential."[46] The sunny disposition of seventy-three-year old Drake and the positive people in our lives is something we can focus on and practice. Let the positives be central to our lives.

Over the past twenty years, research and evidence indicate that caregiving is a major public health issue. Greater degrees of depression and stress are also associated with several factors, such as elder behaviour, functional abilities, cognition, amount of care, relationship with elder, gender, and amount of care needed. Patients or loved ones suffer when caregivers have emotional problems. This just compounds the problems already evident. Why couldn't that negativity be flipped to create positive experiences? There were many times when it could have been easier to be negative with Dad—the times he was short with me, said things that unintentionally hurt others, or just voiced negative thoughts. I remember sitting in a restaurant on one occasion when the waitress wasn't as eager and quick to serve us as Dad wanted. As he was going to say something to her, I interjected and commented on her beautiful name, displayed on her employee badge. I call it the squirrel tactic when attention is diverted from the moment to somewhere else. I borrowed that from the movie *Up*, one of my favourite Pixar films. Or "take the frown and turn it upside down! – an expression from my teacher colleagues.

Research shows that supportive and positive care contributes to a lower mortality rate. Caregiving can be beneficial; it enables caregivers to feel better about who they are, learn new skills, strengthens relationships with others, and creates a positive mindset. Don't we want to feel that "joy" instead of being downhearted?

Recently, I headed off for a few days to visit a relative and just "take my mind off" the everyday little stresses that seemed to be compounded. I also try to ensure that I take time to make someone's "day" with a smile, take flowers or chocolates to Dad's caregivers to say "thanks," and just wake up with a positive attitude! My waking attitude is simply what I choose to think the moment my eyes open, my body stretches into the new day, and my thoughts move me to one word: Thankful. Then I think of all the blessings in my life: breath in my lungs, smell of morning coffee, sunlight on my window, a bird song, and, yes, even the roar of a motorbike down my street headed out for the day … because I know there is life all around me.

When I was helping one of the ladies in Dad's laundry room one day, we were having a discussion about health. She told me that she was blind in one eye from a stroke, couldn't hear so well anymore, and didn't move as quickly as she would like, but that didn't stop her from being positive. Despite her ailments, she cultivated a positive attitude by putting her feet on the floor each morning and saying: "Thank you, God, for another day."

Personally, I'm an advocate of Pollyanna thinking. I journal, read devotionals, and self talk positive thoughts. I tend to see the bright side in most things, which used to drive my family crazy at times. For instance, the day before I was flying to Mexico with my sister for a week, Dad fell and cut his ear and fractured his pelvis. Everyone was upset. I had been a little worried about him being on his own without my daily visits to the seniors' home if I was away too long. As it turned out, he was told that he needed to be in a wheelchair and that the medical staff would be checking on him more often. They tended to his bandage changes and were more vigilant with his care. That's exactly what I needed to hear, and it made my week away less stressful.

Lastly, it's important for caregivers to have "me time" to meditate, pray, or balance the third component of well-being, which is spirituality. Faith, or spirituality, means different things to different people, but when we're dealing with aging, dementia, or illness, spiritual issues become important as we try to make sense of the meaning of life, death, impending death, and certainly aging and caregiving issues.

Richard Wagamese shares an excellent thought in his book, *Embers—One Ojibway's Meditations*. "We approach our lives on different trajectories, each of us spinning in our own separate, shining orbits. What gives this life its resonance is when those trajectories cross and we become engaged with each other, for as long or as fleetingly as we do."[47]

Addressing personal spiritual needs can help with many different situations. Lots of individuals have questions and want to make sense of, cope with, or find a faith in their situation. Throughout our lives, we deal with change, but looking at the positive aspects can alter our thinking. Looking at the bigger picture can even make things look better. Acknowledging that we have doubts about God, religion, or even spirituality gives us an opportunity to seek help from a spiritual advisor, share our doubts with others, or use our faith to help us cope with our many issues, including caregiving. So what might some of those strategies be?

By trying different coping strategies, a person is able to transform their perspective on caregiving. These are a few ideas gleaned from research. Some I have practiced successfully:

- Speaking to a pastor, chaplain, or religious leader can help us make sense of our situation or put our feelings into perspective.

- Using meditation, devotions, or prayer is helpful.

- Talking with others who are going through a similar circumstance with parents and asking how they coped spiritually can alleviate much tension.

- Connecting with a church, religious community, or support group can provide needed comfort.

- Think about positive practices to nurture yourself—a massage, a short holiday, singing and listening to positive messages in music.

- Get connected to nature, the outdoors, and fresh air.

- Find faith in beliefs and meaning as a caregiver by looking at how you are impacting lives.

- Journal, color, paint, or engage in some other form of art.

According to researchers Erin Long and Sari Shuman,[48] four trends were evident in inter-faith communities. They found that faith adds to well-being, collaboration promoted wider participation with the community and strengthened faith, resources were helpful, and creative engagement was successful.

The research does indicate that positive relationships and well-being are attributed to religion, spirituality, caring for others, friendships, and the joy of living. Giving of self takes on many forms. Simple tasks such as walking the dog, being in nature, giving a hug, laughing together, getting a good night's sleep, making dinner, dancing, or even having a good cry are positive actions.

When Mom was in the hospice, the chaplain came to see her, pray with her, and talk with and comfort her when we couldn't be there. Even after Mom passed away, they followed up on us as a family to ensure we were emotionally well. I can attest to the fact that faith, prayer, and support has kept me in strength, sanity, and health for the rougher times I go through. When I come across a photo of Mom and Dad, or my brother, who also passed away, I know that they're not in pain, and that gives me peace. When moments of grief or painful memories consume me, I'm able to pray wherever I am, read scripture, listen to a favourite song, play the piano, or read a book and know that this is life and I will be all right. I remember when I was retiring from a career of thirty-six years, had just lost my brother, and my marriage was breaking up. Shortly after that, I ended up caring for both my parents, but here I am now—a stronger, more resilient woman because of the struggles I went through.

Caring for a loved one can be a daunting task, but there are hundreds of devotional books, inspirational websites, podcasts, and Bible verses that uplift and provide comfort during those times of struggle. One of my favourite verses is Psalm 121:1–2: "*I lift my eyes up to the mountains—where does my help come from? My help comes from the Lord, the Maker of heaven and earth*" (NIV). More often, though, I would refer to Isaiah 40:28–31: "*Do you not know? Have you not heard? The Lord is the everlasting God, the Creator of the end of the earth. He will not grow tired or weary, and his understanding no one can fathom. He gives strength to the weary and increases the power of the weak. Even youths grow tired and weary, and young men stumble and fall; but those who hope in the Lord will renew their strength. They will soar on wings like eagles; they will run and not grow weary; they will walk and not be faint.*"

Mom would listen to her psalms on the CD player in the hospice, and I will often play my songs on the piano or iPad to connect with God. Going to the mountains, singing in church or in the vehicle, reading devotions, taking a walk in the winter, or meeting a friend for a visit helps get others through "those days." Think of what things you could do to relieve your stress. Your health is important, especially if you're caregiving.

You need to find what "fits" for you, your lifestyle, and rhythms. Taking time to address those three aspects of life—physical, mental/emotional, and spiritual— enables you to thrive, not just survive. We can do this! And yes, I'll say a little prayer for you.

CHAPTER 7 TAKEAWAYS:

- ☐ It's important for caregivers to have "**me time.**" (**Spiritual**) *Are you taking time?*
- ☐ Get exercise, eat nutritiously, and sleep well. (**Physical**) *Are you up and moving?*
- ☐ Connect with others and stay positive. (**Mental/ Emotional**) *Have you connected with someone?*

DID YOU KNOW?

You can check out the most recent statistics and quick facts regarding health by googling albertahealthservices.ca

https://www.albertahealthservices.ca/assets/about/publications/ahs-quick-facts -annual.pdf[49]

CHAPTER 8:
A DIFFERENT HOME
(HOUSING FOR THE ELDERLY)
A Home "Away from" Home

"Caregiving often calls us to lean into love we didn't know possible."
Tia Walker - "The Inspired Caregiver" [50]

A few years ago, Mom and Dad and a few of us siblings started the search for an ideal seniors' home that would suit their needs at the time. Mom and Dad had sold their traditional home and were looking to the future. Needless to say, we found many different types of seniors' housing. Some were too expensive. In some cases, the location wasn't ideal, there wasn't enough space, activities were minimal or not engaging enough, or the food plans were insufficient. All the homes were so different and unique. Where were they going to live? Where should they go?

These questions will crop up when the time for living at home is not an option. "Where" may depend on health issues, spousal death, or any manner of end of life circumstance. "When" to start looking is now. Planning can be done with a clear mind and conversation, not to mention mobility while one is able.

Recently, my aunt shared the story of her and a friend.

For a couple of months, my friend Jo and I went visiting some of the senior care homes. We just wanted to know what was out there for us when the time comes, so we could pick out the one we liked the best and hopefully not get plunked down just anywhere.

Well, now we are being bombarded with invitations to various functions. Last evening, we attended an outdoor dance band performance at Missionwood. Today, we were invited to a TEA at Chatstworth. Every week we've gone to some sort of entertainment around the residences. Social Butterflies is what we are.

They are wooing us …

They all think we should move in now, but our plans are to stay in our homes as long as we can with health care coming in … a lot cheaper too. Some of those places are quite ritzy, and I'd have to mortgage my first born to think of moving in there.

There is an array of housing options available to all people, but planning aids in a stress-free, quick process of elimination. Once you've done the legwork, you can have fun checking the various places and even trying some of their meals. According to a website called "Comfortlife,[51]" there's a checklist of questions to ask when you're ready to consider a new home for your loved ones. Chapter three focused on traditional home, hospital care, and hospices, and this chapter pertains to the various types of seniors' homes.

Recently when I spoke to a representative at an eldercare conference, I asked her what advice she'd give to someone searching for a seniors' home. Her answer verified what the research says. Go to the home you're interested in several times, at several different times of the day, and talk to several different staff and residents.

Stay for lunch, check out the facility, and ask lots of questions. Good advice! There will be different staff on during different shifts, and you'll meet different people—or the same ones—each time you visit.

Make a list of the various homes you're interested in. Then when you go for "the tour," you can ask the same questions at each and gather as much information as possible before making any decisions. Even though many of the homes have websites and pamphlets, real conversations and visits enable you to pose questions that arise and need to be addressed face to face. Sometimes it's like going on that vacation that doesn't even come close to the images on the pamphlet or Expedia descriptors! I remember one home we visited in particular. The pamphlet showed a beautiful room with lots of lighting and open spaces, but when we visited, we noticed the drab, unkept carpet, the poor lighting, and the soft smell of urine in the air. Personal experience speaks volumes!

When a decision has been made, it's critical to go over the contract and paperwork and understand the fine print on the documents. Wait a minute … what are those checkpoint questions? Let's group them according to easy categories:

Location of the Building

- Is it near the current neighbourhood where the elderly or caregiver presently live?

- Is it near relatives, family members, or friends who can visit regularly?

- Is it in the city, suburbs, or small town?

- Is it accessible to the bank, grocery store, or other amenities?

- Is it picturesque and easy to get to?

First Impressions do count, and they leave lasting imprints.

Of the Building

- Are the grounds well kept and maintained?

- Do you like the building design?

- What are some of the security features?

- Is it a new or old building—any recent upgrades or renovations?

- Is there easy access, ample or underground parking, including for guests who come to visit?

- Is it tidy? Clean? Spacious?

- Is there a "smell" of urine in the air?

Of the Residents

- Are they friendly and easy to chat with?

- Are they friendly to each other?

- Do you or your elder know anyone?

- Are the residents satisfied? (Be sure to chat with more than one or two!)

- Are the residents content or dissatisfied and why?

- What is the age range of residents?

- What are some of the stories of residents?

- Is there an online website to check some of the testimonials?

Of the Staff

- Are they kind and welcoming when you arrive?

- Do they know the residents by name?

- Are they interested in "life" at the home?

- Are you able to chat with them to get their impressions of the home?

- Will they take time for you to chat informally?

Services and Amenities

- What is offered?

- Is there a set schedule of events daily, weekly, monthly?

- Do they have activities your loved ones would like to be involved in?

- Is there housekeeping? Laundry facilities?

- What range of activities are available at the home or nearby?

- Is there an exercise room? Pool? Common area for games?

- Is there a handicap bus available?

- Are you able to choose which services you require?

- Is there a space to share when others come to visit?

Food

- What is the dining room experience like? *Many homes offer complimentary lunch or supper if you book ahead for a tour.*

- What are the menu choices?

- Can dietary needs be accommodated?

- Can friends or relatives join for a meal?

- Are snacks provided?

- Is there a dietician on staff?

- Can you speak with the chef or kitchen staff?

- What is the average cost for a meal?

- Are meals served by staff?
- Is the food "tasty"?

Health and Medical

- Are the nurse practioners, nurses' aids and LPNs (Licensed Nurse Practioner) qualified?
- Can a doctor come for "house visits"?
- Is there a nurse on call or staff 24/7?
- Would you have to move if health issues or other needs increased?
- Is there a care plan in place for residents?
- Is there a case worker for patients?
- Do the staff distribute medication?
- Is there a pharmacy connected to the facility?
- Do residents wear "call buttons"?
- Is there assisted living?
- Is the facility an L1, L2, L3? (referring to level of care)
- Do they have weekly clinics to check blood pressure?
- Do they have regular "checks" on patients?

The Suite or Room

- Is it comfortable and cheery?
- Is there room for favourite furniture?
- Could you make a snack or breakfast in the room?
- Does it have ample supports such as a wall rail in the bathroom?

- Is there room for a wheelchair or walker?

- Does it have a kitchen?

- Can you decorate and put up pictures?

- Is there carpet, tiles, or linoleum?

- Does it have windows or a balcony?

- Is the washroom "user friendly"?

Wellness

- Are there fitness or wellness classes or spaces available?

- Is there a gym, workout space, or a pool?

- Are there positive messages displayed?

- Are there various positive incentives? (piano player at lunch or a band in the evenings, not just bingo!)

- Is there a walking group or exercise class?

Lifelong Learning

- What kind of classes or courses are offered, such as yoga or painting?

- Are the classes on or off site?

- Are the interests of the residents being addressed?

- What are the wait times for classes?

- Is there a computer available?

- Is there a "fun coordinator" on site?

Volunteering

- Does the residence provide opportunities to volunteer in the wider community?

- What are some of the opportunities within the home to volunteer? (reading, games, puzzles, hymn sing)
- What are the other organizations and resources available in the community?
- Is there a group that come in regularly to volunteer with the seniors?
- What programs are available in the area?
- Have you met any of the organizers or volunteers?

Finances

- What are the monthly costs?
- What are the "extra costs"?
- Are there any subsidies available?
- Is it affordable?
- Is low-cost housing for seniors available (government agencies)
- What is the breakdown of costs per service?
- Is there a damage or holding deposit?
- Are invoices given monthly?
- How are they distributed? (mail or email)

Mom and dad lived in a retirement home for six months to experience life there in case they needed to settle for more care. They met a number of couples and enjoyed many of the monthly events and outings. They even had some excellent meal choices; however, their experience proved to be an "eye opener" for them. Mom did not relish the lack of nutritional food available, as well as dining with the same group of people at mealtime. They also learned that they had to pay for some of the excursions and bus trips, as well as anything deemed "extra" to their care, such as a walker.

After the short six-month stint, they opted to move into a condominium complex to have more independence, enjoy different cooking and meals, and choose their own activities. They received some assisted living; however, they enjoyed that freedom afforded them in their own space. I believe they would have stayed in the senior home a little longer, but Mom was "too young-minded" and preferred not to have the same conversation at each mealtime. She did, however, make many friends and gave suggestions for change, such as a healthier menu and different types of entertainment, that still impacts others there today. Dad was just happy to go along with whatever suggestions Mom made.

When Mom's health concerns grew too great and we had to admit her to a hospice after she returned from the hospital, our planning was a blessing. Because we had done a lot of our homework, checked out various places, got our questions answered, and had a good idea of what care Dad needed, we were able to have Dad on a waiting list at a residence of his and Mom's choosing.

After meeting with the management of the various homes and having conversations with siblings and family, and researching and comparing the different options from all our planning, we were all relieved that Dad was happy with the choice we collectively made, and he was able to move without anyone panicking. It was a smooth transition.

The wonderful aspect about our experience was that the process went smoothly and we were informed that if Dad's dementia should ever increase, or his medical needs need addressing, he could literally move "down the hall" to the other side of the building to get more care. We also had Dad's room "set up," so he simply brought his suitcase and moved in.

This was unlike the experience of one of his tablemates, who didn't have an easy transition and complained of moving boxes and putting up pictures with little or no help. The moving truck simply came and dropped off his furniture and possessions in his room. They had both opted for "independent living." Another couple have family close by, and they are so pleased that they chose to leave their farm and have everyone help them move into the home before they had health issues. Ironically, the husband had a heart attack shortly after they moved in, but he was given immediate medical attention, which saved his life. That would not have been the case had they been living in the country, miles from a hospital or any care. Recently he suffered another stroke, and her health continues to deteriorate.

Be sure to ask about transitions within the building should any medical concerns arise. When my father was finally declining in health, both physically and mentally, we started asking questions about having him transferred to the memory care unit. The process was started, but it wasn't until my dad experienced a traumatic event one night that the staff acted upon what we had been informing them of. Dad needed more care, but apparently, he had other medical issues that needed addressing. He wasn't going to be able to just "move down the hall." We now had to work with Transition Services to find dad another "home." Even though we had "planned" on having Dad stay in the same building, our choice was made for us based on his medical condition. This will sometimes be the case, and the medical staff and doctors will determine next steps.

Predictions for 2051 are that the number of senior housing options will have quadrupled from our present number in 2019.[52] That's only thirty years from now! Navigating the vast array of options can be a complex endeavor; therefore, the need for pre-planning becomes even more important so that families can make well-informed, confident choices ahead of time. Even if it seems silly at the time.

Each province in Canada has resources and options available, but there are basically three to four levels of housing.

Independent Living is designed for active, healthy seniors who do not need assistance. These places range from luxury condos and senior apartments to 55+ Communities and Adult-Active Retirement Communities. These are paid for privately and can range from $1,500–$4,000 CAD per month. Some of the complexes have activities and events each month, caretakers and groundskeepers, or even gated entries. You can find these facilities in most towns, cities, and even out of country.

The next level, similar to independent living, is Assisted Living. Many amenities such as meal-services, housekeeping, and medication supervision are provided, as are things like assistance with compression stockings or other forms of personalized assistance. The need for future assistance is possibly anticipated. This supportive housing, congregate, or retirement care often charges a flat rate for basic services, and prices range from $1,600–$5,000 CAD a month depending on services used.

Other factors to consider when looking at housing are location and type and size of residence or apartment. These facilities are generally larger and cater to a large group of seniors who call this their "home." Some of these homes have been recently built or renovated, and some are in ill repair. Check them out in person, as you will be thankful you did!

My father was in this type of facility and quite enjoyed the camaraderie of the table group he sat with for meal times, the Thursday evening jam sessions and hymn sings, and the monthly birthday cake parties for the residents. He also had LPNs who assisted him with his compression socks, distributed his medication, and brought him meals if he wasn't feeling up to going down to the dining room. Each complex is unique with its own schedules, regulations, and services.

The third level of housing is classified as Private or Government Subsidized Residential Care Homes. Many of these facilities offer short and long-term care and fill the gap between independent living and nursing homes. Some of these places even specialize in memory care. Depending on the health issue or services needed, costs can vary greatly, with dementia care alone costing even more. Again, each facility or company has information regarding what is available and at what cost.

With Alzheimer's or dementia care, treatment is generally provided in a secured area to prevent patients from leaving the building or getting lost. We were thankful that my grandmother was moved to this type of facility after she was found during the dead of winter walking with no coat down the main street of her little town. Luckily, one of the town workers knew who she was and got her back to the home without any frostbite! Many of these facilities also have qualified health care workers who are trained to care for these diseases. Because prices tend to be greater, ranging from $3,000– $7,000 CAD a month, there's a need for higher level care to ensure the residents' safety.

Some buildings, like the one my father resided at, incorporate all levels of care. The Alberta Health Services website provides ample information that explains different levels of care and facilities.

Long-term care is for people needing 24-hour medical attention. In addition to medical care, these facilities offer a range of amenities and services. Often an application form must be completed to determine the level of care that will be needed. These are often filled out by a doctor after a patient visit.

Again, Alberta Health Services has more information, forms, and guides to help individuals make informed, wise choices and decisions for their loved ones. Being proactive and exploring what's available is always a good option, or you could end up like Wayne Greggain. He was living at Sechelt Hospital as recently as June of last year (2018), unable to walk and sliding into dementia, but not because he needed treatment.[53] He's not famous, but he represents many who are waiting on residential care for a room in a facility. Stories on the news like his are becoming common.

Even as far away as Australia, aged care specialists are saying that the average age of seniors entering senior care homes is approximately eighty-three. They suggest that people start thinking about planning for this future need in their fifties and sixties.[54]

The bottom line is that as our aging population requires more care, we do not want to fill our hospitals with seniors who could be quite comfortable living in another type of housing more suitable for the care they need. All it would take is some pre-planning and research of what is available based on needs. Because these statistics are constantly changing, one needs to be prepared to make changes in the future.

There are also other items to consider when "checking out" facilities:

- Check the length of waiting lists. (Is there a deposit?)

- Check websites for facility reviews. (Look for complaints and posts.)

- Visit the facility a number of times at different times, as staffing changes.

- Talk with a variety of residents (or their family members) about the experiences of living there.

- Ask for licenses or copies of inspection reports.

- Find out how family members are kept informed.

- Ask them to explain how medical emergencies are handled.

An explanation from the staff regarding how they handled medical emergencies would have been helpful to me at one time. I had just finished supper when my cell phone rang.

"Your dad has had a fall. We've called the ambulance and they're on their way. He cut his ear and head and will probably need stitches. Our RN has assessed the situation and feels that this is treatment he'll need at the hospital."

"So what do I do?"

"You're welcome to meet the ambulance down at the hospital. It should be there in about ten to fifteen minutes."

I was on my way, confident that everything that could be done at the moment was happening and that my dad was in good hands. I was thankful he had pushed his "green button" from the medical alarm on his wrist!

Having that connection or communication with your loved one's facility workers keeps you and others informed when you can't be there to address various concerns or emergencies, as in my dad's case.

Living out of province is even more onerous on the caregiver, and reliance on the senior home staff is even more valuable to keep up to date with progress or decline of your loved one's health. Regular phone calls or emails keep you connected and informed.

The staff of these facilities often want the family or friends to be involved in the lives of their residents. Recently, they had a pancake breakfast and a rodeo afternoon with fun games for the seniors. It was enlightening to see the various staff members interacting with the seniors and encouraging and supporting them in their endeavors to shoot the pop cans with the Nerf guns and throw the rubber chicken into the hula hoop. Many facilities partner with local community organizations to ensure that residents have a good quality of life. Many of the facilities hire a recreation manager to coordinate various activities throughout the day, week, or month. Recently, the facility my father lived in added quilt making, with the seniors giving back to the community by donating the quilts to the women's shelter. Both groups benefit from the interactions.

In the larger centres or cities, some non-profit groups are eligible for funding, but in the rural communities, staff have to be more creative. At a few facilities, staff have even hosted dances in which the bus picks up seniors at one home and brings them over to another facility so they can mingle. They'll often take seniors to events in the community as well, or host things like a Spring Ball where participants can interact on a weekly basis. Some facilities are using university students to live with and assist seniors at the homes as compensation for their rent. Breanna Massey, a twenty-two-year-old university student, decided to write the life story of a senior living in a retirement residence for one of her assignments.[55] She found it very rewarding, and the senior and his family were thrilled.

The bottom line is that there are many choices offered to seniors. As our aging population increases, demand, availability, and affordability will continue to be factors determining where our loved ones spend their winter years. Hopefully they are healthy, happy, and safe. And then when their "time has come," the last home they will visit will be the funeral home.

We want what 's best for our loved ones. We want them to be comfortable, and we want less worry and stress in our lives. We can start making good choices before things "go south." We can do this!

CHAPTER 8 TAKEAWAYS:

- ☐ Make a **list of the various homes or facilities** to visit.

- ☐ Ask the **checkpoint questions from this chapter** when you **visit** the various facilities.

- ☐ When a decision has been made, go over the contract and **paperwork** and understand the fine print on the documents.

DID YOU KNOW?

Fact: Canada offers some of the best retirement homes to seniors who are able to afford them.

Fact: In a 2015 report, "Future Care for Canadian Seniors: A Status Quo Forecast," the Conference Board of Canada estimated that by 2026, over 2.4 million Canadians age sixty-five and over will require paid and unpaid continuing care support —by 2046, this number will reach nearly 3.3 million.[56]

CHAPTER 9:
THE FUNERAL

The Final Days

"It behooves me to remember as I advance in age that death is an inevitable part of the life cycle rather than a medical failure."
Lisa J. Shultz, "A Chance to Say Goodbye: Reflections on Losing a Parent"[57]

The grieving after losing a loved one, the heartache of loss, the celebration of a life well-lived are all ways that a person may react after one we loved has passed on. We have no way of preparing ourselves emotionally when the time comes to say goodbye. For caregivers, there is sadness and perhaps anger, guilt, or confusion. Some may see it as a blessing, especially if their loved one was suffering at the end of his or her life. Sad to say as well, some families are excited about the prospect of being beneficiaries to large estates. Whatever the outcome, losing a family member or friend will affect someone, somewhere, somehow.

According to Dr. Jody Carrington, more people are opting not to have a service, ceremony, or closure after their death. "The person making the decision to not have a funeral or celebration, should not be the only one in charge of that decision because the purpose of ceremony is for those of us left behind.[58]"

When we can openly and honestly discuss death and dying, we understand that our life is limited and we can make a difference as a caregiver at the end of someone's life. Because death is so unpredictable, it's difficult to know how death will happen, but we can sometimes prepare for it when it does.

The process of dying could take days or even years. Pre-planning the funeral or memorial service, preparing for bereavement support, planning the division of the estate, and even having the obituary and eulogy written can all ease the stress of the days following a loved one's passing. Recently I attended a celebration of life service for a colleague who had suffered from cancer for many years. When he knew he was near death and ready to accept that fact, he was able to talk with his minister and arrange most of his funeral. Unfortunately, he was in much pain and not thinking clearly, and in the end, his family decided much of the arrangement for his memorial service.

By making arrangements ahead of time, caregivers can ascertain their parents' or elders' preferences prior to their death. Not only are the logistics taken care of, as well as the loved one's wishes, but pre-planning a funeral or memorial service reduces costs considerably. Why have unclear heads and heavy hearts when dealing with all the funeral arrangements in the midst of mourning?

One tip is to review funeral plans yearly, just in case the ownership of the funeral home changes or it closes. As well, check the price variations on funeral homes, so everyone is kept informed in case of the need to revise the plans. This way, if a funeral home closes or relocates, you will find out sooner rather than later.

During this stressful time, there are important decisions to be made, and not everyone may agree on cost, let alone what the loved ones would have wanted or requested at their death. Being involved in the planning is a gift to the living and gives a sense of relief to all involved. Mom and Dad were in their seventies when Mom was diagnosed with cancer the second time. That's when they made arrangements with the funeral home near their residence. Experts from Alberta Health Services suggest having things in place by aged sixty-five, as previously mentioned.

At one of our family gatherings, my nephew was visiting from out of town. At the supper table at my parents' house, my mother, being quite religious, asked my nephew, "Do you know where you're going when your life is over?" Mom was expecting a heavenly reply.

In response, my nephew retorted, "Yeah, I'm going to Frank's Funeral Home!"

Nonetheless, no one is required to use a funeral home for planning or hosting the funeral, but staff can serve as valuable people for consulting and taking care of a number of details that will need to be addressed. There are countless decisions to be made, and often they can guide the caregiver and loved ones in decision making.

A few places in the United States actually offer free pizza for people to come in and pre-plan their funerals! It is a business. A dying one at that.

So, what are the planning steps in the event that someone wants to prepare for death? Just like there are lots of choices for where one wants to live as a senior, there are lots of choices to make regarding life after death. The following is the beginning of a list:

- For the final resting place, will the loved one be buried?

- Cremated?

- Entombed?

- Or have their body donated for research or organ donor service?

- Will there be funeral services?

- A memorial service?

- Cemetery service?

- Religious service?

- Who is going to give the eulogy should one be required?

- What will we say in the obituary?

- What are the names of the papers where we send the obituary?

- How much is it going to cost to have it in the newspapers?

- Do we have to contact someone to lead the service? Should there be one?

- Does the church/facility require money for the use of the space?

- What are all the items we need to address if there is a memorial or a funeral?

- Other questions that will arise …

Many individuals don't realize that death notices, obituaries, and burial permits require payment, not to mention all the costs incurred before, during, and after the funeral for various facilities, caskets or urns, or even thank you notes for all the pallbearers, just to name a few. As well, because the remains need to be deposited, provincial regulations must be followed. It's all the little items that many people are not familiar with or have no desire to know about beforehand that add up.

When Mom passed away, miles from their prearranged funeral and resting place, we had to have her body transported to the burial site for the day of the funeral. That was an added cost. We also had to decide what she would wear in her casket. What were we to do with her glasses? Who would sing at the funeral? What church would we use? Thankfully, Mom and Dad's pre-planning arrangements made things less stressful, because we had a number to call and most of the details were to be taken care of by the prearranged funeral home. We just had to answer their questions and they took over. Thankfully, my sister still lived near my parents' burial site. There were fewer details to take care of because arrangements had already been made. The funeral home even took care of stationery needs such as Thank You cards. Because my parents had attended a church for a number of years, the ladies' group provided the coffee and refreshments after the funeral, and the church family assisted us with all the arrangements in conjunction with the funeral home—from the PowerPoint presentation and music to the pallbearer instructions at the graveside.

My siblings and I had time to grieve with loved ones and celebrate our mother's life in a private ceremony at the graveside prior to the service without feeling rushed, stressed, or frenzied to get things done. Most of us lived in other cities and provinces, so it would not have been easy to make all the arrangements as smoothly as things had gone. We were also thankful that we had that positive ending to Mom's life, because little did we know that within the year, we would be standing by that same gravesite and saying goodbye to Dad.

So, what can you do to alleviate many of the difficult decisions ahead of time? Because I live in Alberta, I would use websites that cover: decisions before death, planning a funeral, final resting place and after the funeral with lists and forms. There are various resources for other provinces as well.

Because many people don't know where to begin, who to turn to, or even how to get started after someone has passed, pre-planning funerals offers the opportunity to control all the details before-hand—even financially and, to some extent, emotionally. You can have that peace of mind knowing that you will be remembered the way you wanted to be, so talking with that funeral director can get you started on arrangements and they can at least give you an idea of what details need to be taken care of either before or after a death. Depending on what town or city one lives in will determine what resources are available for you. Note that there are differences in price between funeral homes as well.

Because Mom gave me the photos for the slide presentation, the songs she wanted sung, and had even asked the singers ahead of time, we didn't have to agree on or discuss what "Mom would have wanted." After Mom's death, I asked my father what songs he would like sung on "his day," because we needed to start thinking about his arrangements for when his "time came." Dad said to me, "Play 'Home on the Range' if you like!" But I knew from talking with him what his favourite songs were!

When Dad passed away, we decided that a graveside service was what he would have wanted. Because the church wasn't available and there was no clergy available, our family arranged the time at the graveside. Sometimes a quiet, personal way to say "goodbye" is something everyone can agree on when the loved one hasn't indi-cated what sort of farewell they want. Again, that communication between family or friends is essential to carry out final wishes. It also helps the people saying goodbye to have closure.

Another thing to note is that "guaranteed pre-plans" lock in prices, so that even if prices rise over the years, there is no cost rise in your premiums for the services you requested. The only cost we incurred when Mom and Dad passed away was the transporting of their bodies, as it was further than the original place of residence.

Other items to note are that you can pay for coffins, chapel, dressing/casketing, staff for services, embalming, basic service fees, and floral or stationery arrangements. Cemetery expenses are also prepaid for graves, headstones, burial containers, and other fees. Checking and comparing various funeral homes and what they offer is similar to the process used to find a home for loved ones.

Basically, the three steps to plan for end of life are as follows:

1. Find out as family members or as caregiver whether prepaid arrangements were made or not. It would be unfortunate to discover, after paying for an expensive funeral, that it was already taken care of.

2. Consider a funeral home near your loved one's "final resting place" and go over details with loved ones regarding any packages they have. In some places, they will even take care of the paperwork after a loved one has passed.

3. Make as many of the funeral or memorial arrangements ahead of time as you can. It will save heartache, disputes, and money problems. Everyone will benefit in the long run.

According to an online poll from the *Globe and Mail*, only 9 per cent of Canadians have planned their funeral.[59] Perhaps this is because the topic is fearful. People don't want to think about their death, or perhaps it's too costly and finances are used for other things besides death, even though we know it will eventually happen.

Dori Denhem knew she wanted to be cremated, so she ordered an urn, selected a location to have it stored behind glass, and decided on a casket for the viewing. She told her kids about a new investment she made recently made.

"I bought a new piece of property. It's got a glass door. I can see out, and I got a good price on it."

When her kids asked her where it was, she replied, "City View Cemetery."

She was thrilled that she had done something meaningful for her children and had spared them unnecessary grief, frustration, and economic burden. Her children were grateful for what she had done.[60]

The reality is that we will not live forever, so why not understand that life is fleeting and we can make positive impacts through our decisions while we're living. Pre- planning also accounts for knowing what lies ahead after a loved one has passed.

Billions of things could happen that you haven't even thought of yet. The question is not whether they will happen. Things are going to happen.[61]

When dealing with the loss of a loved one, you get distracted and consumed with funeral arrangements, the settling of affairs, and dealing with grief. Not only are you now needing to notify others of the death, but you have to tie up all the loose ends of documents, estate, finances, property, and tax returns … not to mention caring for yourself as caregiver and your family.

The wonderful news is that if you have pre-planned, the paperwork will be in one place, the legal documents would have been completed, you'll be aware of the financial situation, you would have communicated with those who need notifying, you'll have the support network available, and you'll be healthy and capable of taking care of the details. It makes sense to have done the ground-work. You can do this!

You are a caregiver! Enjoy the time with loved ones and make memories in those last days. When your time comes, details will have been arranged for you, so that your loved ones can rest in peace as well. Having that plan in place is worth the time at the end of a life. They will be saying a prayer for you.

CHAPTER 9 TAKEAWAYS:

- ☐ Complete **paperwork,** gather legal documents, and establish finances. *When do I take care of all those details?*

- ☐ **Notify** others of the arrangements. *Who do I let know?*

- ☐ Take **care** of yourself. *Am I making sure that I am okay physically, mentally, and emotionally?*

DID YOU KNOW THAT?

Fact: The law gives the executor the right to make the funeral arrangements, not the spouse, family members, or others.

Fact: Even the deceased's wishes can be overridden if his or her wishes are unreasonable? (Imagine having the ashes of cremation scattered over the temples in Thailand at midnight with a helicopter!)

Fact: Grave markers or headstones are NOT included in funeral costs.

Fact: If you do not want to be executor, you can renounce or refuse to act by filling out a form.

Fact: As executor, you will have to pay for any loses out of your own pocket if you fail to carry out your duties properly, and you could be liable.

Fact: Hiring a good estate lawyer will enable you to look after every aspect of the loved one's estate.

Fact: There are two types of assets that do NOT require probate (joint with right of survivorship and designated beneficiary).

Fact: Probate is based on the size of the estate and the province you live in.

Fact: The one debt that takes priority over almost all others is to CRA (Canada Revenue Agency) Not a big surprise! [62]

CHAPTER 10:
REFLECTIONS

One Day It Will Be My Turn

"Another year, another page. A million moments melt away.
The ticking-tocking hands of time; What's found and lost,
remains sublime.
The details that we hold so fast, are nothing more than memories past.
For love is all that lingers true, the bond that ties my heart to you." [63]
Feeding My Mother - Jan Arden, December 29, 2013

Dad was getting worried that he would have to move from his independent living quarters, as his dementia was worsening. He kept referring to the other section of the building, which offered more care medically and mentally, as the Funny Farm. I tried to reassure him that everything was going to be okay and that he was in wonderful hands with the staff and their care for the elderly. After all, I was over there almost every day and had gotten to know the workers better all the time. The friendliness shown to Dad and our family from the residents, the loving hugs and the encouraging words and reassurance of care was evident from many of the staff. We tried keeping Dad as independent for as long as we could.

But I did have to chuckle when we went for our regular Sunday afternoon drive and he asked me where I was taking him.

"A visit to the honey farm—not the Funny Farm, Dad."

It did evoke a smile from him. I smiled inside because I knew that he remembered.

Thankfully there are many seniors who are active mentally, physically, and emotionally and live out a full life of health. Feel blessed, because that's not always the case—the remembering, the smiles, the outings, the health can suddenly or gradually change. In a day, a month, or a year.

I am now able to give advice to my friends who are dealing with many of the same issues and circumstances that I went through. When I tell them that I empathize with them and offer them encouragement, they truly know that I do care and understand, having been through much of it myself. Just as they are transitioning, I did too.

When Dad started telling stories about the old days like he was there, and filling up his garbage cans to water the horses, I realized that we were starting to move into a whole other area of care—memory care, as health workers refer to it. These are the dementia and Alzheimer's patients; the disoriented and sometimes discouraged, irrational, and aggravated elderly; the elderly who have forgotten where they are in the present, but have so many memories from the past. That was another chapter of my life, and there was much reading, research, and discussion to take care of as I watched Dad continue to make sense of the world he was in, not to mention his deteriorating health.

Moments like early one morning at 5:00 a.m. when he called me and my two brothers.

"Who's picking me up at the hotel? I want to go back home!"

We reassured him that he needed to get some sleep and we would see him soon. Or when he fell and cut his hand and he couldn't find the Band-Aids to stop the bleeding—blood everywhere in his bathroom.

When he ended up being transported to two hospitals in one day and couldn't understand where he was. In his final days, when he wondered why Mom, who had passed away ten months before, hadn't come to visit him.

"Do you think she worries about me?" he would ask me.

"Yes, Dad. She loves you and is waiting for you to come home."

I tried to smile, get my exercise, visit with my friends, keep family informed, and hopefully not complain too much about my "life being on hold" as I wrestled with my role as a caregiver.

I did receive beautiful bouquets of flowers and roses from my brothers now and then, as well as daily inspirational messages from my sisters. I got texts and phone messages of encouragement from my friends, colleagues, and church family. Dad had even mentioned at one time that I should be "retired" and not look after him so much.

And as I reached down to fix his shoe lace, I would just say, "Who else better to care and love you, Dad, than one of your daughters?"

I continued to take one day at a time; after all, that's all we really have. I asked the good Lord to continue blessing me with good health after caring for Dad, who did not get any better with his shortness of breath and aching knee and stomach problems. And now that Dad has finally passed away in his sleep and I mourn the loss of him, Mom, and my role as caregiver, I realize that there will be others to love and care for. We can do this! I want to start thinking about a plan for the end of my life so that it will be easier for my children when I'm ready to pass on. But for now ...

I am a caregiver, along with so many others. So many stories.

I recently came across a blog called: *Brutally Honest Memoir on Caring for Aging Parents—A Place for Mom* by cartoonist Roz Chast, which simply reiterated the need for planning. She wished that she could have found joy in caring for her eighty-three- year-old mother. She felt that she had been thrust into this role, and because she was an only child, all responsibility fell on her. She gave up her job and basically her life to care for her mom. She wished that there had been a plan or even time to prepare for all that caregiving entailed. Her advice to others is to plan ahead. She says:

> You WILL get old and don't blindly assume that your child/ children are just joyfully waiting in the wings to take care of you. If you are fortunate enough to have a child that wants to perform this duty, great, but not everyone wants to have this responsibility put upon them all because you didn't plan ahead. This is the most difficult and exhausting process there is. PLAN AHEAD.[64]

So basically, it's that simple. Plan to plan ahead. In this age of complexity, simplify your life. What a better way to do that than start those discussions and conversations, get organized, gather your "tribe," and start researching, gathering and compiling information, and check out what's available. You'll be thankful you did. I can attest to that fact from experience.

As I was gathering information for this book, chatting with friends going through similar circumstances as caregivers, and reflecting on my own life, I realized that I needed to get my plan in order. I have since purchased a small filing box with coloured files. I have sorted through important papers and filed them in the correct place. When I was at the physiotherapist's office this morning filling out paperwork before my appointment, I realized that I needed a list of all my surgeries and their dates to keep in my phone for future references. I also showed my son, who is the executor of my estate, where the safe is with the important papers, and we fiddled with the combination until we got it open!

As I look back on the valuable lessons my parents taught me when they were alive, I realize that even in their deaths, they are still teaching me valuable lessons. I know that my book is a guide for me, my children, and many others who are given the title: caregiver. I pray I can bless someone, a family, a caregiver by encouraging them in some way on the journey. We can do this, as I say a little prayer for you!

CHAPTER 10 TAKEAWAYS:

☐ "Understanding the benefit of planning ahead is sometimes a challenge. Whether you think that one day you may have to be a family caregiver or you are already actively caring for a loved one and feeling the stress of caregiving—planning takes time. Planning will be one more thing on a long list of things to do. However, the time spent planning now can give you more freedom to act later, easing both the burdens and the stresses of family caregiving."[65] *taken from The Family Caregiver's Manual by David Levy, JD, Gerontologist.*

☐ *You should have a healthy relationship with death and it should not be one of fear …*

Death is an ultimate reality of life. The Untethered Soul - Michael A. Singer

CHAPTER 11:
RESOURCES

Where Do I Get All That Information?

COMMUNITY RESOURCES

Trish and I have endeavoured to provide a complete and comprehensive list of options for seniors. These listings are for Calgary only. Some locations outside of Calgary are listed on the websites in this chapter; however, if you're out of province or country, you may have to research your own websites and resources to generate your own lists.

For a more detailed listing of housing, care, and services for seniors, the following websites contain a wealth of useful information.

- https://www.calgary.ca/CSPS/CNS/Pages/Seniors/Seniors-Programs-Services.aspx https://www.albertahealthservices.ca

You can also obtain a free copy of the Seniors Directory of Services produced by Kerby Centre and the City of Calgary, available on most newsstands and at community, health, and seniors' centres.

PRIVATELY OWNED AND OPERATED SENIOR LIVING

Privately owned and operated senior living communities are just that—privately owned and privately paid. Private facilities are typically on the luxury side of the senior living scale and provide a variety of choices in accommodation, programs, and services. Occupancy is based on availability. All facilities, whether private or public, provide tours to prospective residents and their families. It's good to look at a number of residences to be sure you're making the right decision for this stage of life and beyond. Many facilities offer a multitude of programs, services, and levels of care, including independent living, assisted living and dementia care, complex care, respite care/and or trial stays.

You should expect a pre-admission, health assessment, and evaluation. This will help to determine what level of care potential residents will need. What can happen is that a potential resident may believe that they're a good candidate for independent living when in fact their needs would require an assisted living situation. The health assessment and evaluation ensure that all potential residents get the care and level of housing that keeps them well cared for and safe.

AGE CARE

www.agecare.ca

Glenmore 403-253-8806

Midnapore 403-873-2600

Seton 587-349-8444

Sky Pointe 587-619-9000

AMICA MATURE LIFESTYLES

www.amica.ca/

In Calgary operates: **Amica at Aspen Woods** 403-240-4404

ASURA HEALTH

http://asurahealth.com/

The Journey Club, Westman Village

CHARTWELL SENIOR LIVING

https://chartwell.com

Colonel Belcher 587-287-3937

Eau Claire Care Residence 587-287-3943

Fountains of Mission Retirement Residence 587-287-3945

Harbours Retirement Residence 587-287-3941

Royal Park Retirement Residence 587-287-3939

RETIREMENT CONCEPTS

http://www.retirementconcepts.com/

Millrise Seniors Village 403-410-9155

Monterey 403-207-2929

Note: Some private seniors' residences have a percentage of beds that are AHS funded. This is particularly true for assisted living, memory, and long-term care.

REVERA SENIOR LIVING

www.reveraliving.com

Evergreen by Revera 403-201-3555

Chateau Renoir by Revera 403-255-2105

The Edgemont by Revera 403-241-8990

McKenzie Towne Retirement Living 403-257-9331

Scenic Acres Retirement Living 403-208-0338

Bow Crest Long Term Care 403-288-2373

Mount Royal Long Term Care 403-244-8994

McKenzie Towne Long Term Care 403-508-9808

SIGNATURE RETIREMENT LIVING

https://signatureretirementliving.com

Rocky Ridge Retirement Community 403-930-4848

UNITED ACTIVE LIVING

https://unitedactiveliving.com

Garrison Green 403- 685-7200

Fish Creek 587- 481-7907

VERVE SENIOR LIVING

www.verveseniorliving.com

Lake Bonavista Village 403-258-1849

The Lodge at Valley Ridge 403-286-4414

The Prince of Peace 403-285-5680

Trinity Lodge 403-253-7576

ORIGIN SENIOR LIVING

https://www.originway.ca/

Swan Evergreen by Origin 587-481-6638

Whitehorn Village by Origin 403-271-2277

BAYBRIDGE SENIOR LIVING

www.maisonseniorliving.com/specialcare/about-baybridge-senior
-living

Maison 403-476-8992

PUBLIC SECTOR SENIOR LIVING

There is an application process in public sector senior housing operated by AHS (Alberta Health Services). Where possible, clients are placed in one of their top three selections when a bed becomes available. **NOTE:** In some extreme cases, a client may be placed in the first bed available, depending on immediate need. At that point you can choose to be put back on the waiting list for your favoured location, to be moved when there is availability. Communicating with the case worker is necessary to ensure choices are based on need, health, and availability.

AGECARE

Age Care.ca

Age Care is a private senior serving company that also has AHS funded beds, but operates independent living, assisted living, and dementia care housing and care options. Independent living is private pay; the other two are funded by AHS.

BETHANY CARE SOCIETY

www.bethanyseniors.com

Bethany Care Centre (North Hill) 403-284-6000

Bethany Harvest Hills

Bethany also offers a number of affordable housing options.

CAREWEST, A DIVISION OF ALBERTA HEALTH SERVICES

http://carewest.ca/dir/our-centres/

Carewest is an umbrella organization of Alberta Health Services. Carewest is Calgary's largest public care provider of its kind and one of the largest in Canada.

Carewest C3 Beddington 403-520-3350

Carewest Colonel Belcher 403-944-7800

Carewest Dr. Vernon Fanning Centre

Carewest Garrison Green 403-944-0100

Carewest George Boyack 403-267-2750

Carewest Glenmore Park 403-258-7650

Carewest Nickle House 403-520-6735

Carewest Royal Park 403-240-7475

Carewest Rouleau Manor 403-943-9850

Carewest Sarcee 403-686-8100

Carewest Signal Point 403-240-7950

COVENANT HEALTH

www.covenantcare.ca

Dulcina Hospice 587-230-5500

Holy Cross Manor 587-230-7070

Marguerite Manor 587-955-9788

EXTENDICARE

https://www.extendicare.com

Cedars Villa 403-289-0326

Hillcrest 403-249-8915

INTERCARE

www.intercarealberta.com

Brentwood Care Centre 403-289-2576

Chinook Care Centre 403-252-0141

Kingsland Terrace 403-291-0499

Southwood Care Centre 403-252-1194

AFFORDABLE HOUSING FOR SENIORS

SILVERA FOR SENIORS

www.silvera.ca

Silvera for Seniors offers affordable housing with some care options at twenty-two locations across the city.

Subsidies are based on monthly income. Accommodation fees are in effect in all AHS funded facilities.

SUBSIDIZED INDEPENDENT LIVING

(Placement based on monthly income)

http://www.shalem.ca/shalem-campus/

Shalem Haven

Shalem Court (life lease)

Shalem Manor

403-240-2800

Every effort has been made to provide a complete listing of the senior living residences and options in Calgary. There are others that may not be listed here. For more in-depth information, pick up a copy of the Seniors Directory of Services published by the Kerby Centre and the City of Calgary.

A few helpful resources that offer those checklists when you are visiting the various homes are:

- Alzheimer Society Canada

- Advocacy Centre for Elderly—based out of Toronto

- Concerned Friends of Ontario

- Citizens in Care Facilities

http://www.seniors-housing.alberta.ca/documents/Saying-Farewell-Dying-Process-G uide.pdf

COMMUNITIES IN AND AROUND EDMONTON AND CALGARY AND LETHBRIDGE

http://www.comfortlife.ca/retirement-communities/alberta-retirement-homes http://www.agecare.ca/community/agecare-columbia/retirement-living/

https://www.alberta.ca/ministry-seniors-housing.aspx

So, WHEN THE END IS NEAR ... WILL YOUR LOVED ONES KNOW WHAT YOUR FINAL WISHES ARE WHEN THE TIME COMES?

For a list of documents you will need, consult the following website or a lawyer who specializes in wills and estates.

https://www.albertahealthservices.ca/cc/Page15483.aspx

REFERENCES:

https://www.forbes.com

https://vanierinstitute.ca/snapshot-family-caregiving-work-canada/

https://www.ncbi.nlm.nih.gov/pmc/articles/PMC4848186/

https://kurtismycfo.com/

http://www.who.int/mediacentre/news/releases/2015/
   older-persons-day/en/

http://healthydebate.ca/

https://www.albertahealthservices.ca/assets/info/acp/if-hp-acp-
   what-do-I-do-with-mygs.pdf

http://www.promatura.com/about

https://www.letstalkhealth.ca/palliativecare/stories/65-ill-decide

https://www.albertahealthservices.ca/info/Page14778.aspx

https://www.cma.ca/sites/default/files/2018-11/the-state-of-seniors-
   health-care-in-canada-september-2016.pdf

https://www.bankofcanada.ca/unclaimed-balances/

https://www.mclaughlinfinancial.ca/e-newsletter/2014/2014-08/
article-2.htm

https://www.aplaceformom.com/planning-and-advice/articles/
canada-seniors-housing- guide

https://www.alberta.ca/funding-seniors-organizations.aspx

www.passportforwellness.com

www.everydayhealth.com

https://www.alberta.ca/funding-seniors-organizations.aspx

https://www.calgary.ca/CSPS/CNS/Pages/Seniors/Seniors-
Programs-Services.aspx

https://www.albertahealthservices.ca/info/service.aspx?id=1050323

https://www.cma.ca/En/Lists/Medias/the-state-of-seniors-health-
care-in-canada-sept ember-2016.pdf

http://www.who.int/management/quality/assurance/QualityCare_B.
Def.pdf

https://www.youtube.com/watch?v=v2oQC2Mh
L58&list=PLi1tOF1I5ZoW9jvEutpdEw5m
atrJEkLEb&t=0s&index=7 p://eldercarecanada.ca/

https://www.albertahealthservices.ca/info/Page14907.aspx

ENDNOTES

PREFACE

1   https://vancouversun.com/news/local-news/
canadas-first-dementia-village-to-open-in-langley-next-year

2   www.statcan.gc.ca

3   https://www.youtube.com/watch?v=v2oQC2MhL58&list=PLi1tOF1I5ZoW9jv
EutpdEw5matrJEkLEb&index=7&t=0s

INTRODUCTION

4   https://www.brainyquote.com/authors/lou_holtz

5   https://www150.statcan.gc.ca/n1/pub/89-652-x/89-652-x2013001-eng.htm

6   Summit Magazine- Spring/Summer 2018 - page 38

7   Anne Lamott - Traveling Mercies - Some Thoughts on
Faith https://www.penguinrandomhouse.com/books/97402/
traveling-mercies-by-anne-lamott/9780385496094/

8   Rosalynn Carter, former First Lady of United
States of America https://www.nextavenue.org/
rosalynn-carter-pioneering-caregiving-advocate-says-more-must-be-done/

CHAPTER 1

9   John F. Kennedy stated in the State of the Union Address in January 11, 1962

10   p. 28 - Summit Magazine - Mount Royal University - Spring-Summer 2018

11   Gail Sheehy, world renowned author of fifteen books, including Passages in Caregiving - Turning Chaos into Confidence, p. 15

12   Daren Heyland, a professor at Queen's University- an intensive care physician in Ontario

13   J.R.R. Tolkien - The Hobbit quote

14   https://irpp.org/research-studies/supporting-caregivers-and-caregiving-in-an-aging-canada/

15   https://www.brainyquote.com/quotes/lao_tzu_137141

16   http://www.qelccc.ca/

CHAPTER 2

17   High River Times (February 2, 2018), an article entitled, "Death Cafe - A first for High River Community" https://deathcafe.com/deathcafe/6141/

18   https://spiritualityhealth.com/quotes/home-place-you-grow-wanting-leave-and-grow-old

19   https://www.ncbi.nlm.nih.gov/pmc/articles/PMC4848186/ - World Health Organization

20   https://www.albertahealthservices.ca/

21   https://secure.cihi.ca/free_products/hctenglish.pdf Canadian Medical Association study

22   http://www.who.int/mediacentre/news/releases/2015/older-persons-day/en/) http://healthydebate.ca/

23   http://www.advancecareplanning.ca/acp-news/national-ipsos-reid-poll-indicates-majority-of-canadians-havent-talked-about-their-wishes-for-care/

24   https://www.albertahealthservices.ca/assets/info/acp/if-hp-acp-what-do-I-do-with-mygs.pdf Green Sleeve

25   Sheehy, Gail. 2010. Passages in caregiving: turning chaos into confidence. New York: HarperCollins. Page 327

26   http://www.promatura.com/about

27   https://www.letstalkhealth.ca/palliativecare/stories/65-ill-decide

28   www.elderindustry.com

29   https://www.goodreads.com/quotes/600-wrinkles-should-merely-indicate-where-the-smiles-have-been

CHAPTER 4

30   https://www.goodreads.com/quotes/18064-kind-words-can-be-short-and-easy-to-speak-but - Mother Teresa

31   White Springs Journal – September 3, 2018 – Clean, Funny Senior Citizen Jokes – "Hospital Regulations"

32   https://www.cma.ca/sites/default/files/2018-11/the-state-of-seniors-health-care-in-canada-september-2016.pdf

33   https://www150.statcan.gc.ca/n1/pub/89-652-x/89-652-x2013001-eng.htm

CHAPTER 5

34   https://www.aplaceformom.com/blog/time-youre-80-youve-learned-everything/

35   www.legalwills.ca

36   http://www.aclrc.com

CHAPTER 6

37 https://www.goodreads.com/
quotes/43475-the-great-thing-about-getting-older-is-that-you-don-t

38 https://www.bankofcanada.ca/unclaimed-balances/

39 https://www.mclaughlinfinancial.ca/e-newsletter/2014/2014-08/article-2.
htm

40 https://www.aplaceformom.com/canada/how-to-pay-for-senior-housing (2017)

41 https://www.alberta.ca/funding-seniors-organizations.aspx

42 https://globalnews.ca/news/4259206/
nearly-half-of-canadian-seniors-have-financial-worries-report/

43 https://www.helpguide.org/articles/abuse/elder-abuse-and-neglect.htm

CHAPTER 7

44 https://www.brainyquote.com/quotes/celine_dion_457520

45 https://www.msn.com/en-ca/health/wellness/exactly-why-you-keep-waking-up-in-the-middle-of-the-night-according-to-doctors/ar-BBQOLa8?li=AAggNb9&o
cid=mailsignout

46 Drake, Tim, and Chris Middleton. 2009. Six steps to staying younger and feeling sharper. Harlow: Prentice Hall Life.

47 Wagamese, Richard. 2016. Embers: one Ojibway's meditations Page 38

48 https://atapestryoflove.
com/2017/03/07/4-trends-in-building-successful-communitiesof-care/

49 https://albertahealthservices.ca

CHAPTER 8

50 https://www.goodreads.com/author/quotes/7240133.Tia_Walker

51   https://www.comfortlife.ca/

52   https://www.aplaceformom.com/blog/2013-8-27-future-senior-care/

53   https://vancouversun.com/news/local-news/
five-months-in-a-hospital-waiting-for-residential-care

54   https://www.news.com.au/finance/money/why-a-late-start-to-aged-
care-planning-can-be-costly/news-story/42801defcc17610fa3001e432f355
40b

55   https://globalnews.ca/news/4188816/
students-and-seniors-living-together-in-calgary-retirement-home/

56   https://www.conferenceboard.ca/e-library/abstract.aspx?did=7374&AspxAut
oDetectCookieSupport=1

CHAPTER 9

57   https://www.goodreads.com/
quotes/8571138-it-behooves-me-to-remember-as-i-advance-in-age

58   Carrington, Dr. Jody. 2019. Kids These Days: A Game Plan for (Re)
Connecting With Those We Teach, Lead and Love. Printed in Alberta, Canada.
Page 105

59   https://www.theglobeandmail.com/globe-investor/personal-finance/house-
hold-finances/you-cant-cheat-death-but-funeral-preplanning-eases-the-hardship/
article4502744/

60   http://www.whypreplan.org/real-funeral-planning-stories/funeral-preplan-
ning-positivity.php

61   Singer, Michael A. 2007. The untethered soul: the journey beyond yourself.
Oakland, CA: New Harbinger Publications

62   https://www.cma.ca/

CHAPTER 10

63   https://amiesbookreviews.wordpress.com/2018/01/10/feeding-my-mother-by-jann-arden-a-must-read-by-this-multi-talented-canadian-icon/

64   https://www.aplaceformom.com/blog/5-6-14-memoir-on-aging-parents/ - Roz Chast

65   Levy, David. 2016. The Family Caregiver's Manual: A Practical Planning Guide to Managing the Care of Your Loved One. Las Vegas, NV: Central Recovery Press

Printed in Canada